To Aimée, Andrew and Dexter....

Each of you makes me so incredibly proud in your own way. *You* are my reasons to want to keep on breathing. Never forget that for a moment.

"Do you think it matters if they're tiny or deep? he asked. Well, if they're not tiny breaths and they're not deep breaths, then they're just ... breaths. Then you're just breathing for the sake of ... breathing.

... Seize them. Feel them. Love them ..."

– K.A. Tucker, Ten Tiny Breaths

A note from the author

First of all, thank you for taking a peek at my book. When I qualified as an aromatherapist, all the way back in 1993, I never anticipated becoming one of the world's most popular writers about my art. In fact, I never really considered writing at all, and certainly not about breathing problems! But all that changed in 2008 when I had two massive shocks. The first was the discovery of a five week old foetus in my uterus. It revealed itself on the ultrasound scheduling my hysterectomy (15 years after I last gave birth!) The second happened six weeks later when I found myself, breathless, in the back of an ambulance being rushed to hospital with a blood clot in my lungs. These two incidents meant I needed to find a job that I could do quietly at home with a growing baby. I chose to open my precious aromatherapy box and teach people how to use those enigmatic bottles inside.

I found something out that day, in the ambulance. I discovered I really *like* breathing. Until that moment, I had never realised quite how much, in fact I hadn't really ever considered it all. I had taken it completely for granted. Nowadays, whenever an attack of bronchitis takes my breath hostage, it reminds me how scarred my lungs are and of what future might potentially lie ahead of me.

Because here's the thing....

I don't think many people *do* realise how dreadful it is not to be able to breathe, do they?

Perhaps those easy breathers, concentrating on more important things like mobile phones or last night's TV, might have some *small* perception of how their breath affects their *mood*; but do they still know to savour that runner's high, exploding blissful endorphins into their bloodstream, or to register how their breathing becomes shallower in darker moments of panic or fear? How acute is their awareness of how their breath deepens in relaxation, I wonder, and how it slows when they sleep?

People go through life oblivious to how sensual an experience, so full of life, breathing *properly* is. They miss how the whole body moves in an almost indiscernible wave, tipping the head very slightly back as we breathe in, how the chest expands, then the abdomen and the pelvis tilts gently back to receive the air. How it rocks forward as the air leaves our body, relaxing the abdomen, shrinking the chest and flopping the head forward on the exhale. How it utilises the muscles of the neck, the back, the head, the abdomen and intercostals between the ribs. Cough long enough and every one of those muscles will tighten, constrict and invariably start to groan their misuse. You know about them then!

That final descent of breath into the pelvis is the foundation stone of yoga; its energetic caress of the root chakra unleashes sexuality, it grounds and instils self reliance. This almost erotic pelvic emulation of sex, so fertile, betrays the vitality of the journey the oxygen is undertaking, inside. Respiration fires the very processes of life. It fuels our muscles, our digestion, and our thought pathways.

For most people, consideration of breathing is likely to be passing.

Fleeting, nothing more....

Yours and mine?

Well, I find myself thinking about breathing somewhat more. How about you?

I remember how my pulmonary embolism *shrunk* my world. How getting to the toilet was as much as I could do for an entire day. More than that, I recall the terror of making my way, in the cold, to the bus stop to go back to work. I knew coughing was lying in wait, sneering at me, tormenting me to try to beat it into submission, but of course, I couldn't. I knew that too, and I despised it.

I was lucky. The blood clot shattered, thanks to the doctors' medicine, it dispersed and my breath returned to me. But the illness left its mark. The scarring in my lungs, the weakness that always welcomes chest infections with open arms and the certainty that bronchitis is never far away.

Eastern philosophies connect prana, the breath of life with our soul; with our spirit. The rush of breath vitalises us, inspires and invigorates us. It is this liberation that helps us to become the person we were born to be; to live our lives with no limits.

I started this research because I was desperate to regain my spirit; to be free from this panting prison. I wanted to feel relaxed, happy and healthy. I wanted an end to the pain in my chest and my neck. I wanted to fall asleep next to my husband, quietly, without the worry of the sudden explosion of coughing. Most of all, I really wanted to breathe well again.

This is the story that lies behind the words in this book. Fear, and determination to fight the onset of pulmonary disease with every last breath in my body. Bronchitis still attacks, but for short periods now, not much longer than other people suffer with colds. I sing in a choir singing beautiful oratorios, belting out long, sustained top As, and I climb a very steep hill back and forth to school every day. To all intents and purposes, at the moment, respiratory distress is held in abeyance.

Essential oils did that.

It seemed selfish to hold onto the miraculous discoveries that got me to this state of health. So, here are my notes and this is my wish for me, but for you too.

A longer life, with energy and vitality but most of all...hope.

This is my essential oils war on breathing problems....and I *will* win.

Let's rally to arms to gather a fragrant army against this killer that claims so many millions of lives every year.

Come with me...

- Discover essential oils that stop inflammation in its tracks, reduce mucous and clear out debris from the airways and lungs
- Uncover plant extracts proven to work in exactly the same way as the doctor's preferred method of treatment.
- Marvel at how nature has exquisitely created many plants, but particularly eucalyptus, to heal illnesses in the respiratory tract.
- Learn which spice, and usually hazardous oil, influences not only the smooth tissues of the lungs, but also reduces mould spores, dust and pathogens in the environment
- Explore the extraordinary revelations by experts in *psychoneuroimmunology*, about how childhood experiences influence the likelihood of developing respiratory illness...I'll even give you the cutters to sever the chain.

- Identify foods that encourage the body to manufacture mucous and those that make for far happier lungs
- Determine which acupressure points to use to relieve symptoms and calm that wretched cough
- Create aromatherapy blends from recipes designed to improve every aspect of your illness, from breathing problems, to neck pain and even those swollen ankles from your inability to move around.

When you discover just how much evidence there is to prove the diverse ways aromatherapy heals, you will sit there shaking your head in awe. I did, (actually, I still am) and I have been using oils for most of my life.

I promise you there is not another book on the market like this.

It is new paradigm medicine at its very best.

The plants are starting to whisper to us about what they can do. They are surrendering their secrets in laboratories, every day. There is reams and reams of evidence scattered everywhere like a puzzle. I have assembled the COPD jigsaw, and the picture is absolutely astounding.

This is your chance to hear both what the plants *and* the scholars have to say.

Getting the best from this book

When you review the Table of Contents in a moment, you will see it is divided into very clear sections. That said, it has been necessary, sometimes, to sprinkle details about essential oils into the science and data bits. If the stuff about diagnosis, medication, protagonists bores you rigid, that is fine. You can skip it, because every piece of essential oil data is reiterated in the last section. I would however suggest you read the section about the lungs and the emotions.

If you have not already, please take advantage of downloading my free *book The Complete Guide to Clinical Aromatherapy and The Essential Oils of The Physical Body*. This well help you to understand the oils better, to be confident of using them safely and of course, to get your best money's worth out of them as you learn what else you can use them for, outside of respiratory use. I would recommend you also treat yourself to a copy of The Mind Body Spirit of Essential Oils to fully understand the majesty of the mind body connection, but also it will help you get a more comprehensive understanding of some of the science in the emotional sections too

That's the serious bit out of the way....

Now for a couple of not-so-serious comments, before we begin

First, a disclaimer....

Reader, I am English. I live in a cottage, walking distance from an 11th century castle. Being English allows me to hold tea parties when I choose and to be restrained in my use of the word *awesome,* amongst other things. At school, I had spelling tests every week for ten years...I like the way British words are spelled. Sorry! Please, my transatlantic friends - try not to let it bug you too much.

In Texas, Oklahoma and Missouri, you might suffer from *mucus*. Here, in the Shropshire blue and green shed, people can hear me coughing up *mucous* with an O. (Posher? Maybe. I understand The Queen and Prince Charles have also suffered from mucous with an O on occasions when they have wintered at Balmoral!) On really bad days, my phlegm turns a rather delightful shade of my *favourite colour*, green! This grammatical bad *behaviour* is not meant to be malevolent or incendiary. More, know that I have stuck to it with glee. Oh and please, also be forgiving of my rather strange and unusual sense of *humour...*

I can sense someone twitching in Kentucky from here. *Titter titter.*

Lastly

I am not sure you can understand the full beauty of this book, unless you read it with the following in mind.

It is with immense amusement that my family have watched me write this book. I'll let you in on the joke. There are three things in this life I hate.

- Avocados. They taste like soap. Why would anybody eat them?
- Anchovies. They are a joke right? Surely, no-one really wants them a pizza?
- And mucous, snot, slime...

My middle son had a constant dribble down his front as a toddler, as if he oozed ectoplasm from another realm. It didn't help that he would go around telling everyone that he was worried his parents, from the planet Jelly, had forgotten they had left him here. Frankly if I am honest, there was every likelihood that slimy "Ecto" *had* slipped through their webbed fingers and they had rocketed their spaceship away, embarrassed to come back and look for the glistening one. (If you are reading this Mr and Mrs Jelly, he is fine. A little odd, certainly. But fine.) I hoped challenges related to slime were behind me.

Anything vaguely bogey related, snotty or phlegm-y makes me wretch. I can't even say the word "mucous" out loud without recoiling. I thought that *typing* gunky words would be different; easier hopefully. That I would be immune in some way. Like there would be some protective wall between goo and my feelings of nausea and revulsion in thinking of coughing up phlegm.

It seems there is not.

Please know that every time I have typed something vaguely sticky, I have squirmed and said *eeewwww*! Even now I am pulling faces of disgust and leaning away from the screen and these words. Give me puke or blood any day of the week. This whole phlegm thing is like one enormous karmic lesson.

Right then, idiocy over...

Table of contents next, then we will get straight onto the lungs.

Table of Contents

Chapter 1 The Anatomy and Physiology of The Respiratory System

Part of taking control of a disease, I feel, is trying to understand it fully, so you can look at it from many different aspects and assess where things may be going wrong. Breathing is so fundamental to the bodily process, clearly it is going to be complex. The numbers of ways it can dysfunction are many, so first let's acquaint ourselves with its different parts and what exactly it does and why.

The Anatomy of The Respiratory System

Air is taken into the body through two routes, the *primary pathway*, which is via the nose, and the *secondary pathway* where air travels in through the mouth. The nose is full of tiny hairs called *cilia* which catch particles and filter the air. The passageway is also lined with a *mucous membrane*, which helps to warm and moisten the air as it passes through it. Air which has been taken in through both the nose and mouth passes through the nasal cavities into the pharynx. This muscular structure sits at the rear of your throat. It joins the nasal cavities and mouth to the larynx and to the oesophagus below.

The Upper Respiratory System

The upper respiratory system contains the bits, I suppose, most of us would consider to affect a "head cold";

- the nose
- the sinuses
- the pharynx
- the mouth
- part of the throat (larynx) to the voice box.

The functions of this part of the anatomy are to

- Filter and warm the air ready for its passage into the lungs
- Resonate the voice
- Discern scents, smells and tastes and to process them to the brain

Predictably infections of the upper respiratory tract are the most common set in the world, because we count colds, sore throats etc etc. They are miserable, but for the most part not that dangerous. The problems begin when infection progresses further into the body and down to the lower respiratory tract, also known as the lower airway which consists of:

- The lower part of the larynx
- Trachea
- Bronchi
- Bronchioles
- Lungs (including the alveoli)

The Lower Respiratory Tract

From here, the air travels down to the...

Larynx

The larynx is a passage way, made of cartilage, muscles and ligaments. It has three main functions.

- When it is completely open – it allows breathing
- When partially open - it allows us to speak
- When it is closed - it protects the lungs

Trachea

The trachea is a long pipe connecting the larynx to the lungs. Throughout it, there are C-shaped rings of cartilage. Near the end of it, the trachea splits into two: a right and a left *bronchus. (One bronchus, two bronchi)* and they enter the lungs at a point called the *hilam.* Here, the pulmonary arteries also enter the lungs (which supply the lungs with oxygenated air) and the pulmonary veins, which transport carbon dioxide back out of the body.

Bronchi

Once inside of the lungs, the bronchi separate into *lobar bronchi,* also known as *secondary bronchi.* From there, they subdivide further into *segmental* or *tertiary bronchi.* It helps to imagine these like a tree with no leaves, with branches coming off a trunk and then further growing little twigs off them.

The function of the lobar bronchi is to supply the different lobes (or sections) of the lungs. The right lung has three lobes and the left one has just two, this in turn dictates that the right lung has three lobar bronchi and the left naturally has just the two.

Bronchioles

So, the journey continues and the bronchi become ever smaller, so they then become *bronchioles*. These are much littler and unlike their larger compatriots, do not have any cartilage. They further develop into *alveolar ducts* and then *alveolar sacs* and finally *alveoli*.

Lungs

Together the lungs weigh just under 3lb, with the right lung weighing slightly more than the left.The lungs themselves are surrounded by a pleural cavity or pleura. This is constructed from serous membrane (serous membrane being two smooth layers filled with fluid). The *visceral pleura* lies against the surface of the lung and the *parietal pleura* lies against the surface of the thorax (or your chest). The *pleural cavity* lies between these two viscera and is filled with pleural fluid. This gap is miniscule and so the layer of fluid is exceptionally thin. You might recognise an inflammation of this area as the painful condition, pleurisy.

Alveoli

Together the lungs contain 1500 miles (2400 km) of airways and 300-500 million alveoli. Alveoli are extremely thin. These sacs of air look like miniscule bunches of grapes. They have a huge surface area and fantastic blood supply to diffuse gases through. Their job is to enable gas exchange, putting oxygen into the blood and removing CO2 via tiny capillaries in their walls. It is thought that if all the capillaries that surround the alveoli were untangled, and laid down end to end, they would extend for 616 miles (992 km).

Throughout the lower respiratory tract, we find these cilia again. This time they are called epithelial cilia. Epithelial tissue is covered thickly by cilia which stand up in tiny finger like protrusions. Their job is to sweep away dust and grime particles. Single cilia are not strong enough to do the job on their alone, so several are recruited to push pathogens along (and through) the mucous which covers the tissue surface.

When we experience a cold or in more severe problems such as bronchitis and emphysema, the speed – **the cilia beat frequency** - of the sweeping is slowed. This reduced work output means gradually there is a build up of "rubbish" in the airways and lungs.

Respiration

The term to respire (as in respiratory), relates to the process which happens when you take in air. It is useful to remember that ***breathing* and *respiration* are not the same thing.**

Breathing in, is correctly termed ***inspiration***, ***expiration*** is how we **expel it** again. **Respiration** is the ***chemical process*** which happens as we do this, as the body takes in glucose and produces energy from it. This energy will be used to power muscles and enable them to contract, and also to maintain body temperature, as well as other functions.

There are two types of respiration

Aerobic respiration requires air, in particular oxygen

Anaerobic respiration does not use oxygen

The chemical equation that happens in ***aerobic respiration*** looks like this:

Glucose + Oxygen = Carbon Dioxide (CO_2) + Water+ Energy

That is to say that that energy is created but there are also bi-products of water and carbon dioxide.

The chemical equation that happens in ***anaerobic respiration*** looks like this:

Glucose = Lactic Acid + Energy

Clearly then, those of us who struggle to get enough oxygen into our lungs create anaerobic respiration more often, and thus manufacture more lactic acid. Lactic acid is essentially a toxin that needs to be removed from the body, but actually this is not very efficiently done. It solidifies, and muscles which are made up of bundles of fibres struggle to cleanse themselves of these sharp crystals. Often you will feel pain as the fibres scratch over them. A common example is that horrid aching sensation, familiar after strenuous exercise. Perhaps some of you can relate to the sensation of your ribs hurting after a time, but also your back and neck from repeated coughing? This is because your body has not had enough oxygen to supply how much your muscles have had to work; lactic acid crystals have built up and are constricting the fibres of your muscles. Massage and exercise can both improve these. In particular, **juniper** oil dissipates lactic acid and **lavender** will soothe the pain)

It is also useful here to point out that in anaerobic respiration there is no water bi-product. As such, you may recognise dry coughing and an arid mouth too.

This oxygen taken in and the resulting carbon dioxide, is transported around the body via the blood. The heart pumps it around, allowing it to deliver oxygen to the cells. It then picks up CO_2 to guide it out of the body through the lungs. It travels around a separate, secondary circuit, the *pulmonary system*, where it drops off the CO_2 and collects more oxygen.

Respiration and the Circulatory System

Blood is made up of four main constituents

- Red blood cells
- White blood cells
- Platelets
- Plasma

Red blood cells

We call these cells, but strictly speaking they are not, because they do not have a nucleus that a cell would more correctly require. They are disc shaped and are slightly concave. They contain a protein called haemoglobin whose job it is to carry oxygen. Their curved surface means they can be packed full of the optimum amount of oxygen possible.

White blood cells

These are fundamental to our understanding of the bronchitis and COPD reaction.

The job of these is to surround infections and viruses in the blood and to overpower them. They defend the body and provide our immunity to illness. They do this by creating *anti-bodies* and *anti-toxins*.

There are far fewer white blood cells than red ones, (about 5 times less) but they come in many differing types. We will explore them more when we think about the infection and inflammation response later in the book.

Platelets

These are tiny fragments of cells controlling the way your blood clots. If you cut yourself then platelets create a scab.

Plasma

This thin, straw coloured fluid makes up the liquid of the blood. It carries glucose to all the cells in the body (which it picks up from the small intestine, where it has been absorbed from food) and also carbon dioxide. It carries the CO_2 back to the lungs where it diffuses across the cell walls and is then breathed out.

Chapter 2 The conditions; their possible causes and protagonists

COPD

Chronic Obstructive Pulmonary Disease is the umbrella term for Chronic Bronchitis, Emphysema and Chronic Obstructive Airways Disease. Each, eventually, over time leads to damage in the lungs. The difficulty sufferers of COPD experience, is mainly due to the narrowing of the airways.

Typical signs of COPD are:

- Increasing breathlessness in times of activity
- Coughing up grey/yellow phlegm
- Frequent chest infections

It is believed there are around 3 million people living with COPD in Britain, but only around 900,000 are recorded, as many people do not seek help for their breathing difficulties, dismissing their symptoms simply as a smoker's cough. In the US it is believed there are 12 million diagnosed and a further 12 million who are unaware of their condition.

Let's look at each condition in turn.

Bronchitis

The first clue to the disease is found in its ending; - *itis* . Any condition ending in ***itis*** is medical speak for an illness involving **inflammation**. Here we find an inflammation of the bronchioles. There are two types of bronchitis. These are *Acute Bronchitis* and *Chronic Bronchitis*.

Whilst the biological mechanism is the same, in that the bronchioles become inflamed, the distinction between them is more to do with the length and severity of the flare up.

The word *acute* means sudden, sharp and unexpected. The term *chronic* pertains to a lingering and ongoing illness.

Acute Bronchitis

Acute bronchitis is usually a feverish condition that may have begun as an infection of the upper respiratory tract and then has found its way down to the lungs. About 10% of acute bronchitis attacks can be attributed to bacterial infections from: *Mycoplasma pneumoniae, Chlamydophila pneumoniae, Bordetella pertussis, Streptococcus pneumoniae,* and *Haemophilus influenzae*.

Acute bronchitis is one of the top five reasons for people visiting the doctor, and one of the most common chest infections. Particularly common in children under the age of five, it often follows a cold and may be accompanied by a sore throat and wheezing.

The cough can hurt like crazy because it begins by being very dry and if you are anything like me, you are driven barmy by this repeated hacking. Over time though, the cough irritates the lungs to create more mucous to lubricate them. This is when you start to cough up the delightful sputum, which can either be clear, pus-filled or sometimes blood stained because you have damaged a vessel with all of your coughing. This process can be encouraged and quickened using inhalations with oils such **benzoin**.

So as acute bronchitis develops, you have this transition from a dry cough to a wetter one which tends to be less painful too, because the mucous lubricates the bronchi. Acute bronchitis tends to last only a few days and will often clear up on its own as the body's own defences kick in, recruit enough warrior cells called macrophages, that can overcome the infection, supress and kill it.

You should seek the doctor's advice if:

- The cough is severe and lasts for more than three weeks
- If sputum and phlegm becomes blood stained or shows traces of blood
- You have a fever of over 38°C – 100.4°F – or above for more than three days
- You have an underlying heart or lung condition (such as asthma)

Chronic Bronchitis

A diagnosis of chronic bronchitis is usually given if symptoms have lasted for more than three months over two successive years. It is estimated there are around 2 million adults living in the UK with chronic bronchitis, most of them over the age of 50. Symptoms do not usually become severe enough to diagnose chronic bronchitis until the age of 35. Women are more than twice as likely to be diagnosed with chronic bronchitis than men.

Chronic bronchitis is often exacerbated by : *Streptococcus pneumoniae, Non-typable Haemophilus influenzae,* or *Moraxella catarrhalis*

Sufferers of chronic bronchitis often find their symptoms become much worse in the winter, and to suffer flare-ups more than continual difficulty breathing. It is not unusual to suffer two or three flare ups a year. Simple adjustments such as wearing a scarf over your mouth in cold weather, can have massive affects on the severity of attacks.

To assess how severe a patients breathing problems have become, the doctor with do tests using a spirometer. He will perform a FEV test (Forced Exhale Value) to see how much air can be expelled in one second, and then an FVC (Forced Vital Capacity) to assess the total amount of air they can exhale. These are then compared with a set value which is taken from an average of other people of a similar age group.

Many people who have chronic bronchitis from long term smoking also develop emphysema. Historically more men than women were diagnosed, however in 2011 the trend reversed. This is most likely due to the popularity of smoking to women. Terrifyingly **female smokers are thirteen times more likely to die** from emphysema than those women who never have.

Emphysema

After long periods of breathing issues, the alveoli or air sacs become damaged. Their tissues are very thin and when they weaken they collapse. In a healthy lung, these air sacs are like tiny bunches of grapes and are able to support large amounts of oxygen. As they weaken and collapse, this leaves a much larger space, which is less efficient in holding and processing oxygen.

The air is supposed to escape, but in emphysema it can get trapped, meaning there is less room for fresh, vital air. Instead, the lungs hold on to stale and less vibrant air depleted in oxygen.

There is no cure for emphysema. Whilst there are treatments which can improve how effectively the lungs work, there is no reversal for the collapse of the sacs.

Allopathic Medicine

The term *allopathic medicine* refers to the care you receive from your doctor. Its definition is to treat symptoms it sees and then to attempt to suppress them. So your medicine may be designed to treat the mucous in your air passageways, reduce your cough or help you get more oxygen into your lungs.

In later stages of COPD, the doctor will likely give you a cannister of oxygen to help you breathe. Earlier on in your illness though, they take two main tracks of therapy. The first is to try to calm the inflammation and for this they use something called β_2-adrenergic receptor agonists. Agonists and antagonists are covered in more depth in The Essential Oils of the Mind Body Spirit, but from the greatest height...

β_2 (pronounced Beta 2) is a receptor, so consider that to be like a keyhole. Ligands are the keys to open the lock and make neurotransmitting cells work. When the process is allowed to complete we refer to the ligand as an agonist. Antagonists are the deadbolt that prevents the ligand from activating the cell. In the case of COPD, *the β_2-adrenergic receptor agonist* smoothes the muscles and tissues of the airways, opening and relaxing them.

Sadly, for many people these drugs have side effects. They stop them sleeping, give them the tremors and increase anxiety. In severe cases they can cause tachycardia and pulmonary oedema.

Frankincense has been found to be an effective β_2-adrenergic receptor agonist, as has **evening primrose oil**. There is a slight codicil with evening primrose in that it only works if a patient is not already taking synthetic steroids (I don't know why). Therefore it is worth reaching for these in the first few days of a flare up before you take the doctor's meds. Incidentally evening primrose can be taken as capsules or as used as a carrier oil. It is not distilled essential oil. (Purely based on intuition rather than any evidence, it seems to make sense to me, to break the evening primrose capsules so the oil trickles down your throat, rather than waiting for gastric juices to absorb and dilute the effects.)

Another treatment, especially in cases where there is prolonged infection, may also be to prescribe steroids. Now, in the short term steroids are mega. You suddenly feel stronger, your symptoms recede and it is seriously happy medicine, but only for a while.

The word *steroid* is a shortened version of *glucocorticosteroid*, which is what the adrenal glands secrete when we are stressed. The process is covered in far more detail in The Professional Stress Solution, but over time the body starts to dysfunction from all the steroids in the body. The adrenal glands become exhausted, they drain power from the liver, pituitary gland and kidneys. After a while cortisol in the system stops being a natural anti-inflammatory, reverses on its own axis, and it actually sets off its own inflammatory response. We will talk about that more when we look at the effects of the emotions on our breathing.

For now...

Oils that support the adrenals (depleted after steroid use) are *mandarin, camomile maroc* and *geranium.*

Complementary medicine, in contrast to allopathic medicine looks at the symptom, treats it and then wants to know "But what happened to cause it in the first place?" After we have addressed the problems of the coughing, breathlessness and pain, then we will look at what may be causing the symptoms on a day to day basis. We try to isolate and treat the source of the problem. It is only by entirely disseminating the illness is it possible to treat it fully.

I use the term *complementary medicine*, rather than the term *alternative medicine*, that you may be more familiar with, deliberately and for two reasons. The first is that any treatment or insights I offer are designed to be used *alongside* what the doctor has given you. I will always be the first to say that doctors are better trained than therapists, if only because they have trained for seven years where we only have to train for one. Having said that, it has been predicted that by 2030, the US budgetary expenditure on COPD will top $42 billion, on direct and indirect costs, and that escalating trend is worldwide. For that reason, promoting self care for patients with respiratory conditions is a high priority directive that comes right from the top of every healthcare administration.

Please *do* take this book to show your doctor then **implement my recommendations into *his* care regime**. Essential oils can only do your symptoms good. Perhaps, in time, the doctor may feel happy for you to come off your meds, but that must be a carefully controlled decision and plan taken between the two of you. **Do not stop taking any medications the doctor has given you, without his prior approval.**

The other reason I use the term is I do not feel essential oils can entirely do the job on their own. They most certainly will help you to breathe more easily. Oils such as eucalyptus are wonderful for opening the airways and tea tree is fantastic for attacking any underlying infection, but again we are talking about *symptoms* here. When we dig deeper though, we might find that diet is making your symptoms worse, or perhaps a bone in your spine might be pressing on a nerve sending signals of irritation to your lungs. As the book unfolds you will see there is not only psychological fallout from becoming entirely cheesed off with being breathless....but fascinatingly, certain patterns of behaviour and thinking might have caused the flare up in the first place. If the root cause is not addressed, then the symptoms will be improved, but of course, not fully get better. Given all these aspects then, we might need help from other disciplines too, nutritionists, chiropractors counsellors etc, and so my medicine works complementary to theirs.

Chapter 3 - Exacerbating factors in COPD

- Smoking
- Passive smoking
- Chemicals and Fumes
- Environmental factors such as air pollution
- Genetics
- Diet
- Socioeconomic Factors

Smoking

I hate to tell you what you probably already know but 85-90% of deaths from COPD are attributed to smoking. Given that COPD is the second highest cause of death in the UK and the third highest in the US, that is a terrifying statistic. Cigarettes contain toxins which cause the lungs to act abnormally as they become more and more irritated as the months go by.

Oxidation

The cells in our bodies are subject to oxidation; that is they degrade over time. If you think of cutting an apple in two, over a period of minutes the fresh green turns to a stale nasty brown colour as the cells oxidise. This happens to all our cells. It is a natural process, but it can be speeded up and also slowed down. Smoking makes it happen very quickly indeed.

Reactive Oxidant Species (ROS) are essential for signalling inflammation in our systems but also triggering immune responses too. Smoking disturbs ROS. It raises their number making it far more difficult for our bodies to overcome any irritation caused by air pollution, fungi, pathogens etc. We call this oxidative stress.

Nitric Oxide

In 1992, Nitric Oxide was named Molecule of The Year by the journal *Science* but it took another 6 years for the scientists who had made the discoveries surrounding it, to be awarded the Nobel Prize for Chemistry. Three parties, Robert F. Furchgott, PhD, Louis J. Ignarro, PhD, and Ferid Murad, MD, PhD were jointly awarded the 1998 prize for their work surrounding the molecule.

Nitric oxide is a neutrotransmitter, (the job of a neurotransmitter is to relay signals from the nervous system to the physiology of the body). It is one of the few neurotransmitters in the body that is a gas. It is found in the tissues of every cell and so there is nowhere in our system that is more than one micron away from a supply of it. Its state as a gas means it can move through the body at a startling speed, far faster than many other neurotransmitters.

Its job, very simplistically speaking, is to smooth tissues. It plays a massive part in the cardiovascular and nervous systems. It is now also understood to play a fundamental part in immunity. It is found in the endothelial tissues (the lining) of each cell and it signals vascular smooth cells to relax so vasodilation can take place. Veins and arteries are filled with this relaxant gas and as Nitric Oxide (NO) is activated, it triggers blood vessels to open, allowing parts of the body to be better supplied with circulation.

It is released into our systems at times of pleasure. The best example of how it works is in sexual function. When a man is pleasured, nitric oxide floods through his system allowing blood to flow more freely and effectively to his penis, engorging it and causing an erection. The same happens to a woman when her clitoris is stimulated, but that, clearly, is harder to see!

Many patients who are admitted to hospital with severe COPD are given NO to help them breathe more easily because it relaxes their airways. As yet, the mechanism of why this works is not fully understood, because trials show that patients with both COPD and asthma, naturally, have increased levels of FeNO (that is exhaled nitric oxide) on their breath, leading to suggestions that this is an indicator of *inflammation* in their lungs. But in the words of my old dad "If it ain't broke, don't fix it" so the treatment process is still used because it works, despite clear insights into the exact reasons why. Incidentally, this gas should not be confused with the delicious canister of laughing gas they give you at the dentist or when you are giving birth, which is nitr*ous* oxide.

Bizarrely, nitric oxide seems to a bit of a double agent, because whist he is certainly one of the good guys *inside* of the body, outside he is about as toxic as you can get. Nitric oxide is connected with air pollution and is a bi-product of engine combustion. As such, nitric oxide in the air could be said to be *indirectly* related to breathing difficulties too!

Part of the reason the work into this molecule garnered such attention from the Nobel Prize committee, apart from its obvious importance to coronary health, was the dogged determination by the researchers to prove that Nitric Oxide was no ordinary transmitter but, in fact, a free radical. Free radicals are one of the few things scientists can say, for sure, slows oxidation in cells.

One of the biggest dangers for a smoker, is the damage caused by oxidative stress to cells means there are far fewer of them to produce nitric oxide to smooth out the walls of the lungs. The damage caused by smoking is irreversible, but **the single best thing you can do for yourself and your illness is to stop smoking and to avoid passively breathing in smoke immediately.** Every cigarette you smoke, from here on in, will make your lungs deteriorate even more.

Passive smoking

Whilst active smoking can be blamed for an enormous percentage of sufferers, there are however many thousands who have never smoked a cigarette in their lives. When surveyed many showed links with having spent large amounts of time around a smoker.

Clearly, children and their tiny lungs are at greatest risk. From the baby in utero, being exposed to its mother's smoking, to children of the age of 12 are worst affected, since their lungs are growing and are so fragile and vulnerable.

Part of the diagnosis of COPD depends on a calculation of a patient's FEV, their Forced Expiration Value. Often a lower FEV can be matched to either smoking or passive smoking in adults, leading to the suggestion that the airways maybe affected by not only active but also passive inhalation.

Chemicals and Fumes

Breathing in smoke from open fires can also often exacerbate symptoms. The dust particles launched into the air are minute but are big enough to trigger an inflammatory response in the airways. Shockingly a massive 1 million people die from COPD connected to *indoor pollutants* every year. A particular problem is for women who breathe in noxious fumes while they are cooking. A large percentage of this figure is located in the developing world where poor ventilation provides a very clear danger, however it should make us more vigilant of ensuring extractor fans are on and windows are open, especially when we are using gas burners.

Environmental factors such as air pollution

Dusts and fumes can be a large factor in many patients' symptoms. In particular many workers are exposed daily to known protagonists such as coal, cotton or grain. Coal miners, rock workers and tunnel workers are most at risk from these factors.

Moulds and Fungi

Damp conditions in houses often cause mould spores to form. These can be particularly dangerous for respiratory illnesses as they set up an immune reaction and cause inflammation.

Diet

This is covered in a section on its own but for some people milk and wheat can often make their symptoms worse.

Socioeconomic Factors

Sadly, the difficulty with this particular set of illnesses is many of the protagonists are more likely to be found in the working classes and clearly economics can make it very difficult for sufferers to extract themselves from lifestyles which cause their symptoms to deteriorate. Damp is prevalent in social housing. Certain types of manual labour expose people to airborne particles. Families huddle around kerosene cookers and then feed on junk food lacking in vital vitamins and minerals. Lack of education into the evils of cigarettes mean people still choose to smoke them.

Genetics

In around 10% of COPD cases there is a link to Alpha-1 Antitrypsin Deficiency which the most commonly known risk factor for Emphysema Type 2. In this condition, there is not enough Alpha 1 Antitrypsin in the blood to stop the lungs being attacked by white blood cells. Symptoms of A1AT are shortness of breath and reduced capacity to exercise. These symptoms do not usually reveal themselves before the patient is about 25, and sometimes they never do. In smokers though, signs are usually clear between 32-42 years.

Emphysema has also been found to have links to a genetic mutation in the protein expression of Elastase-2 and its interaction with A1AT. Elastase is a protein that exists in white blood cells called neutrophils. Together with trypsin, neutrophils attack connective tissue, especially in the lungs. Alpha 1 Antitrypsin inhibits elastase, so if a person is A1AT deficient, there is no way to stop this destructive connection between elastase and trypsin, so the lungs undergo an organic assault. The result is pulmonary emphysema.

Elastase determines the mechanics of the connective tissues throughout the entire body, not only the lungs. This means that people with an elastase mutation also have issues with general wounds not healing particularly well either.

Constituents from essential oils have been found to have wound healing effects, on non-healing wounds, that would normally be associated with the expression of elastase and microbial effects._Citronellal, Citral, Geranial, Geraniol, Thymol and Linalool all have abilities to reduce the toxicity with citral, thymol and geraniol coming first second and third!

This is covered in more depth in the essential oils section.

Chapter 4 - The Connection between the Lungs and The Emotions

Alternative medicine has always proposed there is a link between the emotions and health. This is the fundamental idea of the mind-body-spirit connection, that there is a triangle of influence between the three. Physical health is always dependant on a person being entirely comfortable with what is happening in their lives.

At the end of the twentieth century a discovery was made by scientists, which was to change the face of modern medicine for ever. This was that the sensations we feel when we are angry, jealous, happy etc., are actually hormones and neurotransmitters flushing through our bodies. Not only do they affect the body in the here and now (for example, causing stomach ache, breathlessness in panic attacks and blushing...) but they have the ability to stay lodged in the cells for many, many years to come. This idea forms the basis of my book The Mind Body Spirit of Essential Oils.

Let's start by exploring ancient wisdom's thoughts on the lungs and then come back to the science afterwards.

Traditional Chinese Medicine says that each of the organs of the body is affected by a different emotion. At every moment the body changes diffusing from one emotion to another and, of course, colours and shades of any two. The main emotions we see and their corresponding organs are:

- Anger - Liver
- Fear & Fright - Kidneys
- Grief and sadness- Lungs
- Joy - Heart
- Worry and Pensiveness – Spleen

I imagine many of you might already be silently searching your thoughts to see if you can identify any grief and sadness in your mind. Before you decide, let's explore a little deeper.

We now know that there is always a very strange *external* demonstration of the *internal* communications between the mind and body. The mind is no longer accepted to be a separate entity living in the brain, but instead it is made up of the thoughts and memories that flush through the juices of the body in the form of hormones and neurotransmitters. The mind, then, is now believed to run through the entirety of the body. As such, it might be more accurately described as the *bodymind.*

Coughing and struggling to breathe are thought to be outward representations of how the sufferer has been feeling about life generally, and these negative emotions have caused a flare up of symptoms.

In her book *When the Body Speaks the Mind*, Deb Shapiro gives an elegant portrayal of how the lungs convey our feelings about dependence and independence as well as sadness and grief.

She relates how, when as a baby, you gulped your very first breath. This was your first action of independence in this life. You had taken it by yourself, independent of your mother, and the energetic imprint of that memory would stay in the lungs forever. Since that time your lungs have related to life, through this dynamic, again and again. You breathe in and out, securely knowing you will always be safe to take another breath because that first one had been successful and easy to do. Had you not trusted that was so, you would not have given out all of your breath; you may have gasped earlier and tried to hold more air back in reserve.

That trust becomes important.

When someone begins to *stop* trusting that things will be safe in their life, you may see breathing difficulties begin to manifest. Think here of panic and hyperventilation as obvious outward signs, but these maybe more subtle in the cases of bronchitis or asthma, for instance. Symptoms may also arise as the sufferer experiences an overwhelming sense of distrust, perhaps because they perceive something or someone, (most often their mother,) has let them down. They no longer feel they are safe to depend on that person. These feelings of rejection may continue with them throughout life and as such they may take their breathing reaction with them. I use the word *perceive* because often these slights may not have been deliberate acts of neglect, purely how a small child translated them. Just as often as it may relate to some sort of abuse, it might be the parting of a parent because of divorce or death of a loved one, or even getting lost for a few moments in the park.

As with everything in life, practice makes perfect and success breeds success. If something in life goes well, the mind follows and it expects similar events and challenges will also have good and safe outcomes. So transitioning through change and independence becomes easier with practice or harder to do, if things don't work out as you had planned. In the same way if there were repeated traumas, then this practiced subconscious breathing response may become worse.

Imagine then the effects on a child who had a traumatic birth; if their very first breath was stilted, difficult or forced. How might this affect the way they transition *their* way through life? Might we see *them* as clingy children, frightened of change? Or might that be the result of an over protective parent, terrified of the effects germs will have on her child's lungs? Chicken and egg...which came first: the psychology or the physiology? It's impossible to tell.

The lungs are where you welcome life with open arms or you push it away. Do you choose to live life in its fullness or refuse to cut the apron strings? And of course it is not only parent and child. Remember this is the seat of grief.

"What am I going to do without him?" "I can't face life without her."

Dependance....

Choosing independence can feel like you are leaving them behind.

The difficulty with grief, of course, is it has no rules and rationale. There is no handbook to know how it should look or feel. More than that: it is extremely boring and frustrating to anyone around it. So the widow who has felt she had to be strong for her children may forbid herself the chance to express her grief fully. How many people have been told "You have to snap out of this" and been expected to move on before they were ready. In contrast, did they grieve too long and hard? Because imbalance is imbalance whichever way the pendulum swings.

Dependency is a two way thing, of course. It maybe you perceive someone to be overly dependent on you, suffocating...like you can't breathe!

What about the partner who has suffered violence at the hands of someone she loved; someone she should have been able to trust and depend on? How will she react? What about those endless questions about where she has been? Do they make her feel wanted or caged? Does the possibility of answering questions with no logic make her panic ridden and scared? In fact, what happens to her breath in that very first punch? Does she use it to scream and shout back in anger or does she find a coping mechanism that refuses to expose her distress and pain? Does she show her grief to the world, or does she swallow her pride and hope the pain does not show?

Somehow the lungs are a sad place. They nurse un-cried tears and unexpressed pain and sooner or later, it will all come pouring out. Often a sign of lung imbalance is perpetual sobbing, like a tap that cannot be turned off.

It makes me smile to think back to that original equation we had to of aerobic respiration

Glucose + Oxygen = CO_2 *+Water + Energy*

I always wondered what happened to all that water!!! (Although my little boy says "it's the dragon steam on cold days, silly mommy!") Could the tears indeed come from the lungs, I wonder.

Odd, isn't it?

The bronchi bring air into the lungs and then send old air back out of the body. In Chinese Medicine air represents new ideas. We have this strange correlation with change again, then. You can think of the bronchi like tunnels from the inside of the body to the out. In a physically healthy person the air flows unimpeded through the pipe.

Consider then, on the way through, the air meets a pathogen and it tries to move it into the body, but simultaneously the body goes....errr, no....I don't want to bring dust into me, because it does me harm. The reaction causes inflammation and suddenly you can't breathe.

Now, this time, substitute dust for fear of separation, or needing your mum, or even just change in general, and strangely, the lungs act in exactly the same way....cough, cough, cough.

Shapiro states "*Bronchitis is an infection indicating someone or something is affecting you and it creates inflammation, indicating irritation, soreness, anger, upset all in the areas where you breathe in life.*"

As an aside, what is likely to have been the biggest dependency crutch most COPD sufferers will have had? Cigarettes....

I can't help but wonder if the inflammation comes from not being able to get the feelings out. Emphysema for instance has a problem deep in the lungs. Do the feelings remain there? Bronchitis though, exists in the tubes, which suggests the irritants were met on a journey to somewhere new.

In Chinese Medicine there is a feeling that the air we take into the body is representative of new ideas and the vitality we feel with our connection with life. Natalie Kent, author of my-holistic-healing.com, works with the idea that lung issues might be related to having expended a great deal of energy on someone else (again we have this dependence/independence thing) and that air/energy we are taking in is not satisfactorily invested in ourselves. Certainly I can relate to this whole feeling of being smothered or suffocated with feelings of responsibility for others too. How about you?

Of course, from here, when we are burdened with responsibility and duty, it is rare we have the opportunity to break free and try something new, experience life in its richness ....and so the treadmill goes on and on.

40% of sufferers of COPD are reported to also be suffering from depression.

In a survey about how they felt their breathing affected their lives day to day:

- 51% felt it limited their ability to work
- 70% said it affected physical exertion
- 56% reported difficulties doing household chores
- 53% described how it restricted their capacity to join in social activities
- 50% had difficulties sleeping
- 46% felt it affected their day to day family activities

I'd certainly describe that picture as your spirit being stolen from you, wouldn't you? A very depressing picture, indeed.

But is there a chicken and egg situation here? What came first, symptom...or emotion?

Coughing, (potentially wetting yourself on a regular basis, because of the impact on your pelvic floor), feeling worn out through lack of sleep and constant infection....or could it be that the merry-go-round of always having to think about someone else first....or the fear of facing life's experiences without them...

In my experience, it is impossible to discern. Perhaps they are twins!!! Certainly the two *seem to be born of each other*, and are inextricably linked.

Incidentally we know from the earlier chapter on the physiology of the lungs, they are quintessentially linked with the heart. The two work together moving blood and supplying the tissues with oxygen. The emotions affecting the heart are joy and grief and we will look at this more after the science, in the section about the chakras.

Trauma

Despite these thoughts, these ideas are exceptionally difficult to prove, aren't they? My mum has always maintained I was traumatised at birth when "A big, black nurse hung you by one leg under the tap..." however this is the stuff of familial legend, and nothing more. To this day I have no idea why she was supposed to have done that, and in my head I seem to be remembering myself in a pink babygro with white spots. Since one does not tend to be born fully clothed, or indeed wear the outfit that actually belongs to your younger sister's *most-ugly-doll*, Janet, this kinda proves the point that our memories can be less than reliable.

However...

Studies show that children who suffered traumatic childhoods have an increased chance of developing COPD as well, as other diseases, that lead to premature death. In the UK a study was undertaken of adults who had all been born in one particular week in 1958. Scholars assessed observations that had been made about teachers and parents at 7, 11 and 16. These experiences included situations such as neglect, parents separating, or having a parent in prison, as well as socio economic factors involved in their upbringing. The findings were shocking. The chances of premature death were indeed increased through negative childhood experiences...56% for men and a massive 80% more likely in women.

This echoed the findings of the Adverse Childhood Experiences (ACE) study which was undertaken in 1997, where 17,000 participants contributed data about their childhoods to a California HMO (healthcare maintenance organisation). Their findings were that contributors who had four or more types of adverse childhood events had higher rates of ischemic heart disease, cancer, stroke, *chronic bronchitis*, *emphysema,* diabetes, skeletal fractures, and hepatitis than their non-traumatized counterparts. In the case of COPD, instances were calculated to lead to a risk 390% higher...almost four times as likely to develop it.

I have attached a download of the questionnaire which calculates ACE risk factors for you if you feel you would like to carry out your own self- assessment. You can find this at http://www.buildyourownreality.com/ACE-questionnaire

As yet there are no concrete explanations as to why this trauma might have such terrifying outcomes. Some speculate it might be people learn different coping mechanisms, or indeed do not actually learn healthy coping mechanisms at all.

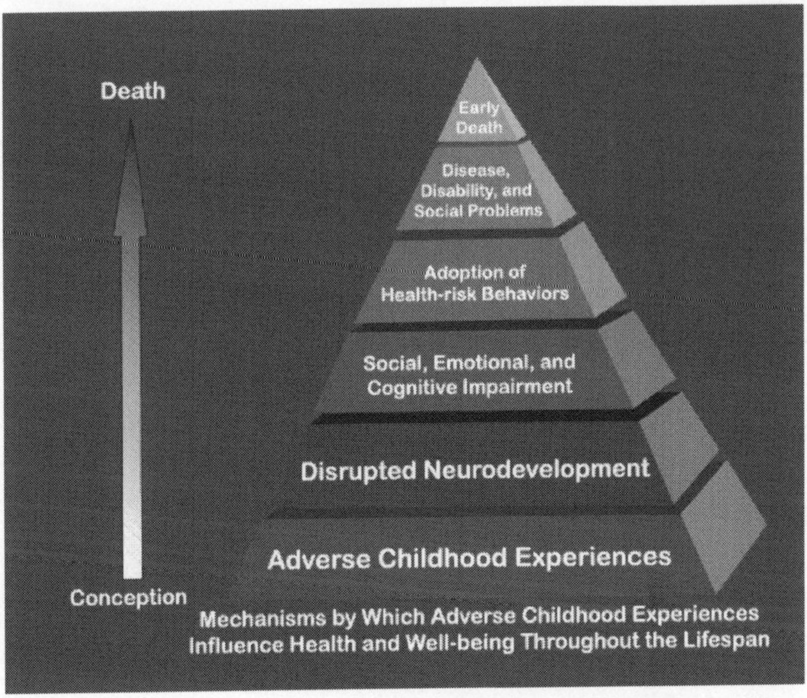

These poor souls are more likely to participate in risky behaviour (and I think really it makes sense to say smoking here, if nothing else) which leads to a deterioration in health.

Another suggestion is proposed, based on the recent finding **that emotions actually control inflammation in the body**. In her paper *Psychological Trauma and Physical Health: A Psychoneuroimmunology Approach to Etiology of Negative Health Effects and Possible Interventions,* Kathleen Kendall-Tackett of the Texas Tech University School of Medicine gives a detailed representation for how this might happen.

Here, she talks of how the emotions cause inflammation in the body. The immune system responds to threats it perceives by sending out pro-inflammatory agents known as cytokines. Their job is to head for the site of physical stress and to inflame it to aid healing. She explains how in their 2005 paper R Glaser & JK Kiecolt-Glaser demonstrated how stresses of both the physical *and the emotional* kind are able to set off this immune response. The cytokines most studied in this context are interleukin-1 (IL-1), interleukin-6 (IL-6), tumor necrosis factor (TNF-), and interferon.

Read that last paragraph again, because you will need to remember it later. It becomes very important.

In my book The Professional Stress Solution I talk a great deal about a hormone secreted by the adrenal glands called cortisol. It is triggered in times of stress and, over time, can become dangerous to our bodily systems. In its normal context cortisol acts as an anti-inflammatory agent in the body, but when it is over produced turns on its head and starts to encourage the inflammatory response by strengthening the actions of IL-1 and IL-6.

In a paper published in September 2014 by Manchester University, findings showed that COPD patients had higher levels of IL6 in their sputum together with a macrophage protein called CCL3. These are both involved in inflammatory actions. It has been suggested that the increased production of IL6 may influence the airway signalling in COPD.

Later in December 2014 Ritz et al. published their findings *in The Journal of Psychosomatic Medicine,* that in laboratory conditions, subjects who had been put under acute stress had elevated levels of FeNO (exhaled nitric oxide) on their breath. Their conclusion: Depressive mood is associated with a reduced mobilization of airway nitric oxide in acute stress.

So to recap that, because even *my* head is spinning with it....

- We know that in times of emotional or physical stress the body sends out cytokines to "heal" the body.
- Cytokines heal by setting up inflammation particularly using interleukins (IL-1 and IL6).
- IL6 in particular is known to be in high levels of the airways of COPD patients and now they have also proven acute stress will elevate these levels.

Just as an aside, in the same way acute and chronic bronchitis are loosely related to how long the symptoms have been lingering, stress is the same.

- The acute stress from the laboratory showed increased levels of nitric oxide.
- Chronic stress will cause the actions of cortisol to "mutate" and make IL-1 & IL6.

Kendall-Tackett goes on to say:

"Depression is not the only cognitive factor that can increase risk of death and disease. Hostility has a similar effect. For people with a hostile world view, life is not benign. People high in trait hostility do not trust others, are suspicious and cynical about human nature, and tend to interpret the actions of others as aggressive (Smith, 1992). This psychological state also triggers the inflammatory response. Individuals who expect the worst from people become hypervigilant to rejection in social relationships, and this world view has discernable, physical sequelae"

(A sequela (usually used in the plural, sequelae) is a pathological condition resulting from a disease, injury, therapy, or other trauma. Typically, a sequela is, in medical language, a chronic condition that is a complication of an acute condition that begins during that acute condition. In ordinary language it may be described as a further condition that is different to, but a consequence of, the first condition.) Thank you, Wikepedia.

So two points to pick up on there, I feel. Trust...we talked about that in the Chinese Medicine section. Could this lack of trust be the difference that changes acute conditions such as bronchitis into more chronic ones, I wonder?

Curiouser and curiouser, said Alice...

Let's think for a moment, about this hostility she describes. It is interesting here, to revisit nitric oxide.

Because of its massive impact on health, scientists are eager to understand exactly how nitric oxide is controlled in the body, not least because it is known to be vital to how serotonin, dopamine and norepinephrine contribute to mood, and physical and mental health. Studies show there is a relationship between nitric oxide and aggression.

In 1995, John Hopkins School of Medicine released findings by Randy Nelson and Sol Snyder into a specially bred strain of mice, created without the genetic marker that manufactures nitric oxide. The male mice had been found to be vehemently aggressive. They perpetually attacked each other and on occasion fought until there were fatalities. They seemed to have no inhibitions and were totally oblivious to sexual rejection from females, continuing with their quests to mate, regardless.

Husband and wife team, Ted and Valina Dawson, had been responsible for breeding the mice and were shocked to find a couple of dead mice, in each set of five, each morning. Since it is very unusual to see mice fight for long, it took some days to realise that, in fact, the mice were killing each other. They were also troubled to note that when male mice were introduced into cages to breed, the females would scream loudly. Soon they noticed that unlike normal male mice, which would mount a girlie when she was on heat, and then leave when she gave no signs of any interest, these would carry on trying to copulate the poor ladies for hours on end despite the mousey squeals and signals of "Will you **** off!"

In every other way the mice were normal and functioned well; in some areas functioned better, in fact. They appeared to be without inhibition, fearlessly approaching physical coordination tasks and performing them better than unaltered mice.

Now, it is important to point out that one of the reasons non-human mammals are used in these trials is because on an evolutionary scale they are identical to humans. Everything about the behaviour of nitric oxide and the neurons is the same in mice as it is in primates. Clearly though, the human mind and physiology is far too complex to say low nitric oxide *is* aggression (or indeed sexual or even *appropriate* behaviour). The number of gene pathways are too numerous and complex for this to be the simple answer but it seems highly likely the two are connected; indeed research is underway to use these mouse findings to pioneer drugs which may be able to help with problems of aggression.

Just to come full circle and sew that section up. Remember nitric oxide relaxes tissues. Its overproduction is indicated in vascular damage in strokes, in heart disease and in COPD. Oxidative stress through smoking reduces the number of cells available to produce nitric oxide, making it harder for smokers to breathe. Indeed treatment of respiratory distress is often treated by relaxing the tissues of the airways using nitric oxide.

Relax....take a chill pill...breathe....

Add to that the statistic that 40% of COPD sufferers are also struggling with the comorbid condition of depression (remember NO is important in synthesis of the mood modulator serotonin) and this low nitric oxide-aggression/hostility connection is starting to feel quite important, don't you think?

So, on the surface it may seem like we should try to avoid negative emotions at all costs; that we should live life as smiley, happy people and all will be well. Wouldn't that be nice? I'd definitely have a pint of that! But a fascinating study into interleukin-6 was undertaken in Japan which shines a slightly different light on the subject.

There has been extensive research into the relationship between negative emotions on IL-6. Findings seem to overwhelmingly agree that its levels are directly related....but only in the West, strangely. In Eastern cultures however, this correlation does not happen so dramatically. An important cultural difference between the two worlds is the way negative emotions are *viewed.* Eastern philosophies integrate all emotions into the human element and welcome them as part of our normal every day experience. They encourage all feelings as fleeting and transient and look to simply allow emotions to change naturally as the seasons of the year would. All emotions are seen as good/normal as long as they are expressed fully and healthily, that they are in balance and are not allowed to veer to the extreme. (*Imbalance is still imbalance, whichever way the pendulum swings.)*

How odd, COPD is the second biggest killer in England; the country well known for its attitude of stiff upper lip and ignoring its emotions.

Clearly, as we start to suffer from the effects of smoking for many years and become annoyed at ourselves, or anger at our dependency on another, or even frustration in being smothered by another...it's fine if we experience these as passing transient emotions but as soon as they come to the forefront of the mind, well then the lungs start to suffer. As Elsa would say from her Frozen tower....Let it go...Let it go....

Post script

To balance the argument, I wanted to confirm if this Eastern philosophy difference meant there was a very low incidence of COPD reported in Japan, but no. Initially statistics *seem* to say yes, but common opinion seems to be the same as everywhere else, that a vast number of cases go unreported. In the same way as the number of bronchitis sufferers in particular, are going up on the female side there, Japan seems also to have far more female smokers. Therefore then, the trend seems to mimic our own.

Chakra Healing

Normally I would put this closer to the essential oils but I think it follows on very nicely from the section on the emotions. The question must certainly be.... "How do these feelings and thoughts find their way to the organs?" Modern medicine now has her own theories about neurotransmitters sending messages from the brain, though the juices of the body, to their relevant parts, and this is addressed at length in Essential Oils of The Mind Body Spirit, as are the mechanisms of the chakras. Therefore it should be enough here to say the respiratory problems, the lungs, trust issues and letting so, all pertain to the heart chakra.

Because I *am* that lazy, I'll just repeat the section from that book for you, but it is worth re-reading it in its correct context in the other book, because it will help you to better understand the joy element, but also the evolution of the energy through each of its stages. It also explains, in detail, how to discern and clearly see the flow of each chakra using a pendulum.

Heart

Located: Centre of the chest

Is aligned to: Love, joy, inner peace

Vibrates on the colour: Green

In health, the energy passes up through the chakras to the crown. As each stage of development evolves so the energy changes, and in fact the wavelengths get higher too. For the heart chakra to function, the wisdom of the lower chakras must have been assimilated. For example if you are aware you are denying yourself feelings, how can you feel joy? If you are feeling like a victim, how can you find peace?

Once the issues of the lower chakras have been aligned then loving energy can fill the heart. Here we feel joy, importantly we can forgive. As we reach the development of the heart chakra we begin to look out of ourselves as to what the world can give. We are open to be loved and are balanced in our approach. This is the time when we learn to [re-]establish trust. Note the association between heavy heart and sadness; the energy pulls the vibration down.

So elements you might look for with this chakra are:

- Bitterness
- Resentment
- Inability to forgive
- Sadness
- Grief

Physical disturbances you might expect to find with an imbalance of the heart chakra are : circulation problems, high blood pressure, shortness of breath, lung and chest complaints, and often you will find the depleted energy sucks vitality through the upper back resulting in pain between the shoulder blades too.

The colour for the heart chakra is green or some people find it more beneficial to meditate in rose pink (actually that always seems to make more sense to me too).

Essential Oils for the Heart Chakra are: *Amber, Basil, Bay, Benzoin, Calendula, Caraway, English Lavender, Galbanum, Hyssop, Lavandin, Mandarin, Mimosa, Myrtle, Ginger, Orange, Parsley Seed, Sage, Spearmint, Sweet Fennel, Tangerine, Thyme, Vanilla, Vertivert, Rose Maroc, Rose geranium, Lime*

Given that, in many people, oxygen cannot be fully pulled down, you may also see problems in the root chakra. I would especially expect to see this in people who have not developed their own independence. Working the root chakra is extremely useful for anyone who becomes light headed, and needs grounding, because of light-headedness from hyperventilation.

Diet

Dairy and Gluten

I found this quite an interesting section because on the outside, it seems strange that food would affect the respiratory system, but there are a few aspects for consideration here.

The first pertains to foods which encourage the body to produce mucous, and as I stated earlier, there are two clear protagonists here: these are gluten and dairy. There seem to be many reports, in particular to people who have removed dairy for a month or so, and found their symptoms to have improved a great deal. I found this right at the end of a particularly horrible bout of "the cough" and removed the bowl of ice cream I had been enjoying (too often) for pudding, and the effect was dramatic.

So, it makes sense to try to swap as many cow's milk products to sheep or goats milk, if you can because they are reputed to be less mucous-making (Charming!)

Clearly for gluten, you need to be aware of bread, pasta, cereals, biscuits and cakes and any wheat related products, but also oats, couscous and many types of beer and chocolate too. Watch out for any sauces and soups that have been thickened, and of course ready meals.

On both counts of dairy and gluten, if in doubt, check the label which must declare them by law if a product contains them.

Salt

In 2011, a study was published which had followed the prognosis of 2183 men in Copenhagen, in a bid to make a final confirmation into a link between salt and respiratory problems. Their findings were a categorical yes, reducing salt intake can prevent chronic bronchitis. Interestingly, those men who reported favouring salty food also had a high likelihood of being smokers, had a high consumption of alcohol and were likely to be exposed to a dusty, dirty environment at work.

Their study goes on to explain how excess sodium can further exacerbate the inflammatory response through various mediums.

Their report concludes:

"The results suggest that salt restriction may prevent chronic bronchitis. The present incidence study supports the idea that high salt intake is not only associated with asthma, bronchial hyperresponsiveness, and various other lung symptoms, but also with chronic bronchitis as conventionally defined. A pragmatic clinical implication would be to include information on salt preference from the bronchitis patient and take action accordingly."

Omega 3

Now, if you went through the section on trauma, calculated your possible prognosis and began to feel very sorry for yourself ...fear not! Solutions are potentially at hand. Research shows there are two things which you can do for yourself which will greatly reduce the impact of the ACE score.

The first is exercise (which we'll cover in a moment) and the second is the consumption of Omega 3.

There have been many studies into the effects of DHA and EPA, the long chain fatty acids, on stress. It seems they are able to moderate and down regulate the stress response. Even modest supplementation caused a significant improvement in mood and the test subjects' attitudes to their stress. Kleicott and Glasier noted in their 2007 paper that patients who had low levels of omega 3 in their diet were more vulnerable to stress but also to illnesses that presented with chronic inflammation. Consumption of DHA and EPA are found to actively reduce the number of cytokines in the system, in particular IL-1, IL3, IL6 and IL10.

Omega 3 balances the affects of omega 6 which are pro-inflammatory. The interesting thing is although the body requires omega 3 to ease inflammation, we do not naturally manufacture it; all sources must come from food.

Sources then:

The primary source is fish, but you would have to be a killer whale to eat the recommended levels of 1.5lbs of fish a day!

Supplementation with *fish oil* is a far better option. You will find it helpfully labelled as Omega 3.

Of course, if you can integrate fish into your diet too....it's all good! Every little helps.

Other sources are **flax seeds, pumpkin seeds, walnuts, beef, soybeans, tofu, Brussel sprouts and cauliflower.** You may recall **evening primrose** being cited as a natural anti-inflammatory (in the beta 2 section)...these effects are thought to come from its high levels of omega 3.

It is all great news for people local to me, in Herefordshire and Shropshire, because our beautiful yellow fields of r**apeseed** are a great source too (**canola** for my US friends, I think). A fantastic reason to buy local!

Naturally, you can integrate flaxseed, rapeseed and walnut oils into dressings and marinades too.

Highest on the fish-y scores are sardines, salmon mackerel, halibut, tuna, herring & shrimps.

Other uses that may be improved by supplementation with omega 3 are asthma, high cholesterol, high blood pressure, arthritis and joint pain, heart disease, rheumatoid arthritis, osteoporosis, diabetes, depression, bi-polar disorder, schizophrenia and cognitive decline. It is also connected with improvement in psoriasis, menstrual pain and IBS.

Honey

Just a little tip as an aside really: A 2012 trial in an Israeli hospital showed that honey seemed to reduce children's coughing allowing them to enjoy far better sleep during their stay.

They were given a single dose of 10g, so 2 tsps of either citrus honey, eucalyptus honey or labitae honey. The trial does not rate any one honey over the other.

Foods which support respiratory health

- Blackcurrants
- Borage
- Carrots
- Chervil
- Figs
- Garlic
- Grapes
- Honey
- Horseradish
- Lettuce
- Mint
- Quince
- Radish
- Sage
- Savory

- Thyme
- Watercress

On days when breathing is particularly difficult, drink infusions of rosemary and borage.

When I have a bad time coughing, I find drinking warm apple juice really helps.

Most of the foods in the above list also have the added benefit of being excellent for detoxifying the body in general. Goodbye manky mucous....you are discharged! No longer required!

Vitamin Therapy

There seems to be opposing evidence. Some says take vitamin C and also zinc. Others seem to say there is no reason to do this. Since both support overall health, I am going to err on the side of saying take a daily supplement.

Respiratory infections can also be an indication of Vitamin A deficiency. Its job is to protect the mucous membranes. Other telltale symptoms are scaly skin and scalp, as well as poor hair health. Spinal infections, dry and itchy eyes can also be clues.

The best possible source of vitamin A is halibut liver oil (fish oils again!), followed by liver, margarine, butter, cheese and eggs. Foods high in vitamin A should be avoided in pregnancy.

Vitamin D3 is particularly important for healthy lungs.

Pulmonary fibrosis, or lung scarring, is improved with selenium and iodine.

Chiropractic

A straight spine is vital to health, since all of the nerves of the body (except for the olfactory nerves which go through the sinus cavity) travel through the spinal column. They are cased within the framework of the vertebrae whose job it is to protect them from damage. These however can become misaligned very easily.

Sometimes it can be a jolt or injury but often simple wear and tear through life can cause them to move. In some cases this can be extremely painful, but often, even though there is no discomfort, the vertebrae may have shifted just enough to rest on one of the nerves. This sends stress signals (including cortisol) to the organs around it.

Now, I have included a download of the spine and the usual illnesses you might expect to see attached to each roaming part. You can find this at http://www.buildyourownreality.com/chiropractic. You will notice when area between T1- T3 becomes misaligned (but especially T3), it is often connected to breathing problems.

The cervical spine vertebrae are also connected with lymphatic drainage, so if subluxtions in this area can prevent the body from being able to cleanse itself properly. This of course will cause build ups of mucous but also the resulting inflammation of the body trying to remove it too.

In some ways this is overly simplistic because the back can be a bit like a domino effect, when one vertebrae moves, another will push the other way to try to compensate and so you get quite a lot of different misalignments going on. In particular you might notice the shoulder mantle being on the diagonal and the pelvis becoming crooked to balance it out.

Doing a very simple check for straightness in the spine, will give you an indicator into whether this might be the source of your problems. Lie down on the bed face down and ask a partner to place their index finger on one side of the spine and their middle finger on the other, so their hand straddles it. Then with very gentle pressure if they trace down to the coccyx slowly, they should be able to discern if any are not quite in line. The diagram also shows what to look for with shoulder and pelvic misalignments.

If this does throw up some clues I would heartily recommend booking in to see a chiropractor because I have seen them do amazing things in a very short amount of time.

Download your chart at http://www.buildyourownreality.com/chiropractic

Acupressure
I can't think of a condition better described as having a blockage of flow really than this. Acupressure removes blockages in the life force qi, promoting better health.

To remove acupressure blockages for bronchitis and COPD, apply pressure to the points illustrated at your free download at http://www.buildyourownreality.com/lung-acu

To begin with you may notice them as very tender. This is a good indicator they need attention. Simply leave your finger gently on their area for about 30 seconds or until you notice the point becoming numb, as the energy starts to flow.

I find there is a great synergy between essential oils and acupressure, so I like to apply oils along the meridian. I have created a diagram for you to download and print off. You will see the lung meridian travels up each arm, down over the main airways and over the chest.

There are many points, some will need work; others may not. You will very quickly become familiar with your own flow. Don't feel you have to work on them all, a couple a day will do, or even just massaging the oils into the meridian may be enough for most.

For clarification, there is an aromatherapy technique called aromatouch, that uses essential oils neat along the meridian.

This is not the same. Please dilute your oils in a carrier before you use them.

Acupressure points which may help to reduce coughing fits are:

Hand

P-9 Right on the tip of the middle finger of each hand

Lu-9 On the front of the wrist, just under the thumb joint

Lu-7 two finger spaces below

Back of the hand

Lu-4 In line with the index finger, level with the thumb joint

TW-3 In line with the ring finger, level with the thumb joint

Foot

The lung area of the foot is located on the fleshy ball of the foot, below the second and middle toe.

SP6 Tender spot along by the side of the Achilles tendon

K3 two finger spaces below

K2 Along the side of the foot, just in line with the front of the leg

Chest

CV22 Just at the top of the ribcage

CV17 just above the base of the sternum

Lu-1 where the breasts meet the shoulders

Of all the spots I find CV22 to be the most effective.

The Importance of Sleep

I get it. I can hear you now. "Easy for you to say..." but sleep is your number one best healing friend.

I can cite a million different papers that extol the virtues of a hearty snooze, but I shall save that for my next book which is about the power of relaxation. In short, sleep down regulates the stress response and reduces inflammation.

I know how hard it is to sleep when you have a cough. I even have a special ugly chair in the living room to spend the night in when I catch the lurgy. It's horrid looking and far too big for the room, but I refuse to risk throwing it out! It reclines so I don't have to lie down and, of course, don't disturb the family.

My mega oils for sleep are yarrow, valerian, lavender and camomile.

You can also try using the free hypnotherapy recording that comes with The Complete Guide. If you haven't yet used it, download it at buildyourownreality.com/free-hypnosis-download/

Breathing Exercises

Many experts will teach you diaphragmatic breathing, which I have found to be very useful, not least because it has helped my capacity to sing. This has double the amount of rewards if the coughing is putting a great deal of pressure on your pelvic floor; perhaps you are struggling with leakage or incontinence. The pelvic floor is part of the same set of fascia as the diaphragm, so when you actively work on relaxing the diaphragm, as you do here, the pelvic floor has chance to rest and recuperate too.

Diaphragmatic breathing

So... to do this.

- Lie flat on the bed or floor and place one hand on your chest and one on your stomach.
- Now breathe in through your nose and out through your mouth, slowly and deliberately three times.

- Now this time focus on your hands as you breathe. I want you to identify which hand or hands move.
- As the air goes into your lungs feel your abdomen expand as it fills with air. Let it grow bigger and as it does feel it lift your hand.
- Now as you expel the air your abdomen should lower taking your hand with it.
- Breathe in again but this time, move your attention to the hand on your chest. If you have perfected the technique, the hand on your chest should not be moving, only the one on your abdomen.

Ideally try to do five minutes of this exercise a day, then try to increase the amount of time. For really excellent pain management work up to twenty minutes. Eventually you will be able to transfer the skill from lying down to controlling the diaphragmatic breathing sitting or standing up.

Think back to what we learned about endorphins in Essential Oils of the Mind Body Spirit too. Breathing deeply releases the natural version of morphine into our systems, as well as reducing the amount of adrenaline and cortisol flowing through our veins.

What's wonderful is you can feel that delicious light-headedness very quickly proving that endorphins are kicking in almost immediately.

This is a great way to give you an extra boost of air, and relax the body too.

Pursed lips breathing

A second school of thought suggests that when you stop consciously thinking about diaphragmatic breathing, the body automatically reverts to a way that is less strenuous on the belly muscles. Gerard Criner, MD, a pulmonologist and professor of medicine at Temple University suggests a better method, especially for sufferers of emphysema might be to learn pursed lip breathing.

- Relax the neck and the shoulder muscles.
- Breathe in for two seconds through your nose. Keep the mouth closed.
- Breathe out for four seconds through pursed lips. If this is too long for you, reduce to breathe in for one second and breathe out for two

Emphysema collapses the airways, but this more controlled method keeps the pressure up in the airways and prevents them from tumbling in. Ideally a patient should learn to breathe this way, as the norm.

Exercise

You may remember that I referred to exercise in that fantastic report by Kathleen Kendal Tackett, as a possible "antidote" to the increases probability of developing COPD from adverse childhood experiences.

She speaks of a two clinical trials that prove exercise is a potent antidepressant, and another that shows it down regulates the inflammatory effects of stress. In the short term, cardio vascular exercise raises the levels of IL-6 (remember him?). Over time though, especially in people with elevated levels of inflammation, cytokines work to lower the levels, inducing an anti-inflammatory effect.

Since older people tend to naturally have higher levels of inflammation (which is possibly why you see COPD in later years) this is a good, reliable sector to watch in clinical studies. One such research project assessed the affects of exercise on 60-90 year olds. They were asked to take a 30 minute walk five times a week, and to walk at a pace that would push their breathing to 60% of its capacity. This testing lasted for 10 weeks.

At the end of the trial, they reported enhanced vitality, a reduction in body pain, improved mood. Their levels of cortisol and IL-6 were all markedly reduced from the readings taken before the exercise intervention.

Authors of a 2007 study also confirmed that inflammation and levels of IL-6 are lower in people who are physically fit and have a lower systolic (upper number) blood pressure reading.

Finally, a 2006 report into diabetic and non diabetic patients showed people who had higher readings of IL-6 also showed signs of cynicism and distrust.

Enough already! The point is made! We need to put our kindles down and get out of our chairs....

As is always the case in illness, the things that are the hardest to do, are things which do us the most good. Give up smoking, and take some exercise. Clearly exercise sounds counter intuitive because day to day breathing is already so difficult, but taking the time to implement these exercises recommended by COPD experts will improve muscle tone and help to improve lung capacity.

Try to do some each day. Daily practice is essential to see progress, but the efforts will pay off.

The emphasis is placed on two specific areas; building strength and building endurance. It is not unusual to see COPD suffers looking almost pigeon chested as their physical frame changes in response to the their illness. In particular, as massage therapists, the most problematic areas we see are tightness in the neck, and also in the chest and upper back areas from all the coughing.

Stretching these muscles not only strengthens the area but also helps to open it up too. If you doubt the effect, then Google pictures of Michael Crawford before and after he became the star of The Phantom of the Opera. As Frank Spencer he was a tiny, weedy little bloke, but all that singing training entirely changed his physique; his upper body became enormous. Possibly there was some upper body work out at the gym, but the diaphragmatic breathing and the growth of his lung capacity had a dramatic effect.

These are simple exercises but are designed to make your lungs work, so expect to get a little breathless. That's Ok. Simply stop exercising for a while. Sit down, relax your shoulders and practice pursed lip breathing, until you feel like you would like to carry on.

There are no prizes for going at it full pelt. Remember, baby steps. Slow and steady progress will ensure you get good improvement in your lung capacity.

Warm Up

Try this sitting or standing, which ever feels most comfortable.

Warm up is crucial, as your muscles and lungs have not been used effectively for so long. Taking time to warm up properly will ensure you don't hurt yourself. Your warm up could be as long as 10-15 minutes.

Shoulder shrugs

Slowly and gently lift your shoulders up towards your ears

Lower down again

4 x up and down

Shoulder circles (arms by sides):

Lift your shoulders round in a circle

Circle slowly and deliberately forwards then backwards

4 x each direction

Head turns

Slowly turn your head as far to the right as you can

Bring it back to centre, nose pointing forward,

Now turn to the left, back to centre

2 x each side

Trunk twists

Sit in a chair, or stand with your feet a shoulder width apart

Fold your arms in front of you

Keep your hips facing forwards and your legs still

Now turn your shoulders only around to the right

Bring it back to the middle, then around to the left

2 x each side

Side bends

Keep your body straight and put your arms by your side

Slide your right arm down your body towards the floor.

Let your hand guide you down the leg

Be careful not to lean forwards

Slide your arm back up

Now repeat on your left side

2 x each side

Knee lifts (hips and knees):

Hold on to a secure surface or sit on a straight backed chair

Slowly lift one knee up to hip level

Don't lift too high

Now lower again

Repeat on your other leg

4 x each side

Heel dig forward

Stand with your hands on your hips

Place one foot in front of the other, place your heel gently on the ground

Bring the foot back to a standing position

Repeat with the other leg

4 x each side

Trunk twists

Sit in a chair, or stand with your feet a shoulder width apart.

Fold your arms in front of you

Keep your hips facing forwards and your legs still

Now turn your shoulders around to the right

Bring them back to centre

Now around to the left

2 x each side

Toe taps to the side

Stand

Put your right leg out to the side and tap your toe on the ground

Bring this leg back to the centre and then repeat with your left

4 x each side

Marching on the spot

Stand tall, standing with feet hip width apart

March on the spot for 1 minute

Endurance /Cardio Vascular Exercise

These exercises build stamina or endurance and they help to keep your heart strong. Do them as long as your breathing and legs will allow you to. Walk or march on the spot at least 5 times per week, daily if possible. Add star jacks and steps or stairs as well on alternating days.

Star Jacks

Stand firmly, holding onto a chair or mantle piece for stability

Take your right arm and leg out to the side at the same time

Bring them back to the centre

Repeat with the left arm and leg

Keep swapping sides, first left, then right, then left again

Take a rest and start again if you get too breathless

Do not forget to sit, relax your neck and shoulders and do pursed lip breathing again to relieve your breathlessness

Try to take a walk out in the fresh air each day if you can. If the weather is bad (ie cold affects your breathing, or humidity too) try marching on the spot, in the house for a minute.

Stand straight and tall and alternately lift your knees to hip level.

Take breathing breaks if you need to and try to resume so you complete one minute a day.

Stair breathing

Taking the stairs each day try to make patterns in your breathing

So:

On set one, breathe in

Breathe out on step two

In on step three

Out on step four

Etc

Feel free to change the pattern as it gets easier, you could try breathe in on steps one and two, out on three and four.

Alternately, just step on and off the bottom step.

Be careful. It's not a race, take your time. Remember you are looking to build strength and endurance. Be the tortoise not the hare!

Static bike/treadmill

Only use under supervision on a low setting. These are very useful and helpful tools.

Cool down and stretches

Please don't skip the cool down; it is every bit as important as your warm up. Remember when we spoke about anaerobic respiration, we spoke about lactic acid? Stretching the muscles helps open up tightness and lets the acid slip away. These stretches will help open up the chest cavity, elongating the fibres of the muscles, making you more limber and stronger.

Feel free to do these in a sitting or standing position. Never force a stretch, only go as far as is comfortable. None of them should be painful- you are aiming for a slight tug, nothing more. Over time you will find the stretch gets longer and easier. Try to hold each stretch for 10-20 seconds.

Back stretch

Clasp your hands in front of you.

Raise them forward, up above your head

Now arch your back so the stretch is even bigger.

You should feel the tug between your shoulder blades

Chest stretch

This time clasp your hands together behind your back

Push your elbows together and let your shoulders open out and move back

You should feel a slight stretch in the muscles at the front of your chest

Arm stretch

Put your right hand on your right shoulder

Lift your elbow upwards

Now stretch it further with help from your left hand

Repeat with the left arm

You'll feel a slight stretch on the back of your upper arm

Trunk stretch

Fold your arms across your body

Keep your legs and hips forwards, and turn your upper body to the right

Hold for a few moments

Slowly return to centre

Now repeat to the left

Side stretch

Place your feet hip width apart

Slowly slide your right hand down the side of your right leg, if standing (or down the right hand side of the chair, if sitting)

In this exercise the stretch is down the left hand side of your body

Return to the starting position and repeat on the other side

Calf stretch

Hold onto something sturdy, like the banister, a radiator or mantle piece

Step one foot forward about 12 ins and move your weight onto it

Try to put the heel of the back foot down on the floor

This is a very deep stretch in the backs of your calf

Repeat on the other side.

Salt and Steam Rooms

We have a salt steam room at our local leisure centre. I find it very helpful for my symptoms. Your doctor may be able to refer you to a centre nearby. (Incidentally if you are thinking of contacting me on facebook.com/TheSecretHealerWrites to ask why salt rooms work when you are supposed to reduce salt in your diet, I'll save you the job. My answer is this...I have no idea. It makes no sense to me either, and frankly it has given me brain ache trying to answer it too.

I feel there is only one possible explanation

It's magic!

OK?

Good.

Crystals

I am not a crystal healer myself, but I do enjoy their energies. According to The Crystal Healer by Phillip Permutt:

Breathing, to ease: Wear a pendant or hold chrysocolla or turquoise. Vandinite can also aid breath control

Bronchitis: Wear a pendant of carnelian, chalcopyrite, chrysocolla, jasper, nebula stone, pyrite, pyrolusite, rutile, tourmaline or turquoise.

He lists crystals for Grief:

Amethyst, angelite, apache tear, aqua aura, bornite, bowenite, dolomite, magnetite, onyx, picture jasper/picture stone, smokey quartz, rose quartz

Insecurity
Agate, angelite, aventurine, boulder opal, labradorite, larvakite, lodestone and muscovite.

Heart Chakra
Malakite

Chapter 6 - Essential Oil Therapy for Bronchitis

The hard part of this is, for many reasons, the thinking does not go in straight lines. For example, later I list cassia as an oil to consider using, because it has can be helpful in many different underlying ways...but actually none of them pertain to breathing! For this reason then, you may possibly find some repetition as I endeavour to make this section one that you can dip into when you need to.

For now we'll start dealing with the most obvious aspects of respiratory illness and then peel back more and more layers as we go...

Respiratory Oils

These oils support and maintain a healthy respiratory system.

- Angelica seed – *Angelic archangelica*
- Basil – *Ocimum basilicum*
- Cardamom - *Elettaria Cardamomum*
- Eucalyptus – *Eucalyptus globulus*
- Ravensara – *Ravensara aromatica*
- Hyssop – *Hyssopus offinalis*
- Inula – *Inula helenium*
- Myrtle – *Myrtus communis*
- Tea tree – *Maleleuca alternifolia*
- Niaouli – *Maleleuca quinquinervia*
- Pine – *Pinus sylvestris*

Fight infection

Clearly this needs to be first line of defence. We will use these oils in both upper and lower infections and try to bash it into submission.

- Elemi - *Canarium luzonicum*
- Cajuput – *Maleleuca leucadendron*
- Niaouli – *Maleleuca quinquinervia*
- Tea tree – *Maleleuca alternifolia*
- Ravensara – *Ravansara aromatica*
- Manuka - *Leptospermum scoparium*
- Kanuka - *Kunzea ericoides*
- Cinnamon – *Cinnamonum zeylanicum*
- Clove - *Syzygium aromaticum*

Induce Mucous

- Benzoin – *Styrax benzoin*

Reduce mucous

- Eucalyptus – *Eucalyptus globulus/ citriodora/radiata/smithii*
- Sweet orange – *Citrus sinensis*
- Lemon – *Citrus limonum*
- Myrtle – *Myrtus communis*

Open airways

- Ginger – *Zingiber officinale*
- Frankincense – *Boswellia carterii*
- Agarwood – *Aquillaria sinensis*
- Eucalyptus - *Eucalyptus globulus/ citriodora/radiata/smithii*
- Peppermint (relax airways) – *Mentha piperita*

Improve tissue elasticity

- Frankincense – *Boswellia carterii*

Help wound healing in emphysema patients

In patients with type 2 emphysema, there is a problem with the expression of a protase responsible for the breakdown of proteins. Constituents from essential oils have been found have wound healing effects on non-healing wounds that would normally be associated with the expression of elastase and microbial effects._Citronellal, Citral, Geranial, Geraniol, Thymol and Linalool all have abilities to reduce the toxicity with citral, thymol and geraniol coming first second and third!

Citral is found in oils of several plants, including lemon myrtle (90-98%), Litsea citrata (90%), Litsea cubeba (70-85%), lemongrass (65-85%), lemon tea-tree (70-80%), petitgrain

(36%), lemon verbena (30-35%), lemon balm (11%), lime (6-9%), lemon (2-5%), and orange.

Geraniol is found in rose oil, palmarosa oil, and citronella oil. It also occurs in small quantities in geranium, lemon.

Oils containing thymol are thyme and oregano.

A plant that contains the most geranial and a large amount of thymol is called *Monarda fistulosa,* a wildflower member of the mint family lamiacaea. There is an essential oil of this, although it is not widely sold. It is a must for suffers of emphysema. Since it smells very much like bergamot, it blends beautifully with eucalyptus too.

Adverse wound healing in emphysema has also been traced to one particular enzyme MMP12 by researchers at the University of Heidelberg. MMP12 is secreted when there is an immune response causing inflammation. Prolonged secretion causes MMP12 to build up and causes damage to the delicate air sacs in emphysema. Boswellia extract has been found to modulate the expression of MMP12 as well as TNF which you may recognise from the section on inflammation. Further studies based in this confirmed the extract to be Boswellia carterii, our belovéd frankincense.

Combat allergens in the environment

- Cassia - *Cinnamomum Cassia*

Improve cilia beat frequency

- Lavender – *Lavendula angustifolia*
- Eucalyptus - *Eucalyptus globulus/ citriodora/radiata/smithii*

And also the carrier oils groundnut/peanut oil and sesame.

Death to Pathogens

In some ways this section is overkill, because you would have to have a pretty tolerant doctor to swab and identify exactly which bug is responsible for your cough. However, I think it is useful to gather a selection of data from which we can create our own needle-free aromatic version of the flu jab. Using a collection of these ensures you fight the germs from as many directions as possible.

My preferred route of healing is always a rub on lotion, but in this case inhalations are useful so you can get the oils to the surface coated by nasties. A 2001 trial showed the most effective way is to use a high concentration of oil for a short amount of time.

You will see horseradish is listed. I have done this for openness because it has achieved brilliant results in lab studies...in a petri dish....not in some poor soul's respiratory tract, thank goodness. Anyone using horseradish essential oil needs to be super, super careful because it is such a vicious irritant; so much so, it is on the International Federation of Aromatherapists hazardous oil list. I think skip the oil and smear horseradish sauce on a beef sandwich. Don't forget to serve with pulmonary carrots!!!! (Just as an aside, the researchers say they believe the oil to be so effective because of the high levels of mustard oils contained in it...what did your grandmother use to combat the irritation of bronchitis and chest infections. Full marks at the back...mustard poultice....which also blistered the skin!)

So here are the oils I have been able to find positive evidence for blasting the bugs.

Mycoplasma pneumoniae

- Bergamot – *Citrus bergamia*
- Tea tree – *Maleleuca alternifolia*

Chlamydophila pneumoniae

No essential oils found but, bizarrely, there seems to be a component in the French cheese, Roquefort, which inhibits its growth!!! Do what you will with that little gem!!!

Bordella petussis

No oils identified

Streptococcus pneumoniae

- Anise – *Pimpinella anisum*
- Eucalyptus - *Eucalyptus globulus / odorata*
- Curry Leaf - *Murraya koenigii*
- Cinnamon – *Cinnamonum zeylanicum*
- Thyme –*Thymus vulgaris*
- Clove- *Syzygium aromaticum*
- Yarrow – *Achillea millefolium*
- Lemongrass - *Cymbopogon flexuosus*

The constituent carvacrol also scored very highly, when it was tested alone. This is found in high concentrations in oregano oil.

Other oils found to help, but which are not commercially available *Monarda puncta, Pinus picae, Juniperus excelsa*

Bieb, Artemisia capillaris (Chinese medicine yin chen, part of the wormwood family) Nasturtian

Haemophilus influenzae

No extra oils to those listed above

Moraxella catarrhalis

- Horseradish - *Armoracia rusticana* (Leave it alone. Nasty oil!)
- Tea tree – *Maleleuca alternifolia*
- Nasturtian - *Tropaeolum majus*

At times chronic bronchitis can also be complicated by infections from *Staphyloccus aureus*

- Agarwood – *Aquilaria sinensis*
- Oregano – *Origanum vulgare*
- Thyme – *Thymus vulgaris*
- Vanilla - *Turnera Diffusa*
- Patchouli- *Pogostemon cablin*
- Ylang ylang – *Cananga odorata*

Oils that have influence the inflammatory response

Through nitric oxide

- Cassia – *Cinnamonum cassia*
- Tagetes – *Tagetes minuta*
- Eucalyptus – *Eucalyptus globulus*
- Thyme – *Thymus vulgaris*
- Peppermint – *Mentha piperita*
- Myrtle- *Myrtus communis*

Through impact on MMP12

- Frankincense – *Boswellia carterii*

Through impact in Beta2

- Evening Primrose - *Oenothera biennis*

Through impact on the gene p38 MAPK-dependent HO-1

This is found to be one of the main reasons for cell migration to the point of inflammation. In cancer it is the protagonist that makes a tumour solid, in COPD is thickens and thus narrows the airways.

- Inula - *Inula helenium*

Treat scarring of the lungs

- Mandarin – *Citrus reticulata*

Oils for the heart Chakra

It is interesting to see these oils in this section. Look how many of them are already indicated for other reasons.

Amber (lifts trauma), Basil, Bay, *Benzoin (induces mucous),* Calendula, Caraway, English Lavender, Galbanum, Hyssop, Lavandin, *Mandarin (helps scarring of the lungs and supports the adrenals),* Mimosa, *Myrtle (anti-inflammatory, anti-microbial, bronchodilator, helps cilia beat frequency, and lovely for children) , Ginger (bronchodilator), Orange,* Parsley Seed, *Sage, Spearmint,* Sweet Fennel, Tangerine, *Thyme, Vanilla,* Vetivert, Rose Maroc, Rose geranium, Lime

Chapter 7 - Documented evidence of the effects each oil has respiratory illness

Basil

Ocimum basilicum

In a 2005 report investigating natural ways to try to treat respiratory infections in the wake of antibiotic resistant illnesses, a Polish contingent explored the possibilities of basil and rosemary oils against the bacteria *Escherichia coli,* which can cause horrible infections in the respiratory tract. Tested against 61 different strains of the bug, both basil and rosemary challenged the bacteria well however basil gave the most effective results. Recommendations have been made to explore the oil more fully, not only for treatment, but also prevention of emergence of new strains.

Basil is particularly good in acute bronchitis because it also reduces fever. A great chest infections hammer all round really.

Safety: Moderate skin irritant, so I would avoid adding to the bath. Not safe for use in pregnancy.

Benzoin

Styrax benzoin

Clears mucous (*Source: Patricia Davis*)

Seems not to be tested in any capacity, but I can attest to it being very good for promoting mucous and releasing you from the hell of that dry cough.

This is a nice one for sore throats too. For little children, stick to inhalations, but if you can bear the taste (and it's not good, trust me) it is a good one to add to your tea tree gargle. 1 drop in a pint of water, (if you are a wuss like me - add an aspirin). And as the actress said to the bishop...*no swallowing, please!*

Hazards: Skin sensitization (low risk).

Cautions (dermal): Hypersensitive, diseased or damaged skin, children under 2 years of age.

Cassia

Cinnamomum cassia

By far the most exciting and terrifying aspect of working on this book has been the recurrent theme of cassia oil. I have a bottle in my box that may potentially have never been opened since I received it five years ago. In fact, that seems very likely since the bottle was still sellotaped secure from being sent through the post. The reason for this, is it is an oil I am slightly scared of. It is a spiteful oil; sharp and very irritating to the skin and mucous membranes. I always give it a wide berth.

But not now I know what I know...

Listen to this!!!!

The first time it stopped me in my tracks was in the research into the section into nitric oxide. You may remember this is involved in the inflammatory response in illness. I was stunned to find that not only were there even any trials into essential oils in this particular aspect of illness, but even more so to find that anyone had even considered cassia....it being so much my friend and all!

In fact, the work had only very recently been done in October 2014 by a team at Chulalongkorn University in Thailand where they tested the effects of both cassia and also an active component, cinnamaldehyde, on the expression of nitric oxide in cells. It was proven to inhibit many different aspects of the inflammatory response. Cytokines, macrophages, cytokines were all adversely affected (through various enzyme expressions). Given that prevention of inflammation was seen in both tests led the scientists to surmise the effective constituent was indeed cinnamaldehyde.

So that was exciting anyway. To discover we hold a potential solution to one of the main protagonists in illness is pretty extraordinary on its own.

But then it happened again.

Scouring my sources to see if anyone had looked into potential oils to combat related strains of mould spores, *Cinnamomum cassia* flashed up again. This time in relation to a strain of mould called aspergillus which is recognised as a severe allergic threat to many sufferers of COPD. A hypersensitivity to the spore can also be a complicating factor in patients with asthma as well as cystic fibrosis.

Is in this trial they identified those who were aspergillus hypersensitive (AH) by giving them a pin prick test. 8.5% of those from the COPD group were identified as being AH, compared to none in the control group.

Most usually the bad guy is identified as *Aspergillus fumigatus*, but it is now decided there may be other rotters in the gang too. *Aspergillus niger* is particular nasty so and so; *Aspergillus flava* is a quieter one, but certainly one you wouldn't want to turn your back on it!

In every case, I was able to find firm evidence of cassia eradicating Aspergillus spores.

May 2013, in Croatia researchers tested patchouli, cassia and Allium tuberosum (garlic chives). Whilst patchouli did inhibit the spores, the concentration used was massive, however cassia showed such excellent results that the recommendation at the end of the report was to try to look for ways to introduce it into food to act as an antimicrobial.

If we go back a few years to 2006, a team in Saurashtra University, India did an extremely large trial into how 75 different essential oils acted on Aspergillus niger. Interestingly, it relates that most of the oils showed some evidence of challenging the pathogen, but the five top (the trial does not list first, second third, sadly) were proven to be *Cinnamomum zeylanicum (bark), Cinnamomum zeylanicum (leaf), Cinnamomum cassia, Syzygium aromaticum and Cymbopogon citrates.* For those of you who have been slacking in your binomial nomenclature class (shame on you!) these are cinnamon bark, leaf, cassia, clove and a strain of lemongrass.

Other oils showing good results in test tubes against *aspergillus* are:

- Thyme - *Thymus vulgaris*
- Basil – *Ocimum basilicum*
- Tagetes – *Tagetes minuta*
- Sage – *Salvia offinalis*
- Cumin – *Cuminum cyminum*
- Pine – *Pinus sylvestris*

Now to quote one of my dad's favourite comedians from my childhood, Jimmy Carson...

"Come here...there's more" (Very broad southern Irish accent is required here, by the way...)

Cassia has also been found to be active against *Dermatophagoides farinae* and *Dermatophagoides pteronyssinus....(*now how's your Latin keeping up?!!)

Not a mould this time.

Far more exciting, and skin crawlingly horrid....

Dust mites.

Specifically *farina,* which is the North American dust mite, and *pteronyssinus*, its (obviously, more chic....) cousin from Northern Europe.

Now to this point I had been struggling with all this a bit because whilst these discoveries are marvellous not only for aromatherapists, but really humankind generally....cassia is still a vicious and cruel oil pretty much guaranteed to give you its very own version of a Chinese burn. So how do we turn this knowledge into practical terms? I most certainly don't want any one of you using cassia on your skin, and I say as much in my *Complete Guide to Clinical Aromatherapy and the Essential Oils for the Physical Body*. Well, the dust mite report opened a whole new realm of thought, because it asserts that the action on the mites has come through fumigation, not actual contact.

Into the air....

In 2012 we received proof from Korea that essential oils were active on airborne bacteria. Therapists have been suspected as much for years and have been merrily making sprays to reduce the spread of flu through the house...but moulds?

I found the proof in a 2009 paper from Tunisia that supported the idea, having used a diffuser containing *salvia offinalis* (sage) to assess whether it could reduce the levels of bacteria, yeast and moulds in the air. Oil was diffused for 5 minutes.

I feel particularly smug to see the best results came from a *smaller* dilution, supporting my ever resounding cry of "**less is more** in essential oils".

The stronger concentration of 1% yielded

54% reduction 1 hour after exposure

55% reduction 6 hours after exposure

55% reduction 24 hour after exposures

0.5% dilution gave a reading of more impressive results of

74% reduction 1 hour after exposure

70% reduction 6 hours after exposure

73% reduction 24 hours after exposure

Despite my smugness, I am however amazed to discover *how* effective it has been found to be, but even more so, just *how long* the effects last.

I later discovered a report from 2006 where similar effects had been assessed by spraying soybean oil throughout a swine house to try to manage its dust levels. Here their tests were limited to 3 hours, and sadly have not listed the dilutions used; but it lists the reduction in dust to around 35%. (Incidentally please note the difference here, this test was on dust, whereas cassia is active on the mites, just to avoid confusion).

Just very quickly, there is another well known fungus which affects the respiratory tract, particularly in cases of pneumonia, called penicillium.

Essential oils found to be active against this are:

- Oregano – *Origanum vulgare*
- Cinnamon – *Cinnamonum zeylanicum*
- Clove - *Syzygium aromaticum*
- Eucalyptus – *Eucalyptus globulus*

Ones found to effective but to lesser degree are:

- Pimento Berry – *Pimenta officinalis*
- Ginger – *Zingiber officinale*
- Thyme – *Thymus vulgare*
- Santolina – *Santolina chamaecyparissias*

What I will say at the end of this is I have experimented using cassia in an evaporator and my breathing definitely improved....but my mood did not. I seemed unable to maintain my usual optimism and ability to look forward and instead became quite dragged down by realities surrounding me. Adding bergamot and lemon to the blend helped a great deal.

Safety data for Cassia oil: Extremely irritant oil. Very burning to the skin and mucous membranes, I would avoid this oil on the skin at all costs. Contraindicated in pregnancy. Inhibits blood clotting. Must not be used with blood clotting or diabetes medications, or at time of surgery. (Safe to use in a diffuser, but I would not want it in an inhalant; too harsh)

Clove

Syzygium aromaticum

Reduces inflammation and increases immunity

Safety: Moderate dermal irritant, so use only in small dilutions. Should be avoided by any patients who have platelet problems such as haemophilia or who are taking blood thinning medication such as heparin, warfarin or enoxoparin.

Eucalyptus

I feel very proud of myself to have tracked down both a 2011 clinical trial and its paper in its entirety, translated from Russian to English! It details a study into children aged 3-4 who suffered from recurrent respiratory illnesses. The major components of the blend they used were eucalyptus and cajeput. It also included peppermint (with the menthol removed), wintergreen, juniper, clove and levomenthol

They deliberately chose oils essential oils which had analgesic, anti-inflammatory, deodorant, antiseptic and antimicrobial action, and could facilitate breathing when the children were cold. Their outcome was a 42.5% decrease in acute respiratory diseases and a 80% improvement in rhinitis.

Of all the oils cited in the book, eucalyptus is found to be the most effective in treating COPD and related bronchial infections. This is primarily because of its high levels of a constituent 1,8 cineole. Much of the safety data you read about eucalyptus and use on children on social networks is utter rubbish. We seem to have created a nanny state about it and frankly it is beginning to make me very angry. Many pages are now stating it is unsafe to use eucalyptus on children under 6 because 1,8-cineole can depress the nervous system and slow respiration.

Yes it can do this; this is exactly the reason it is so effective in bronchitis and the very reason it *should* be used. The correct guideline, according to Tisserand and Young 2013 is do not use near children's faces. Given that there is a mild risk of skin sensitisation, this seems sensible too.

For use on small children please use on their backs or feet. If you are worried about them sucking their toes, then only use on their back. Do not feel concerned about using in a diffuser; this is safe around children too. One drop is adequate and will effectively help to alleviate symptoms.

A 2014 trial at Bonn University in Leipzig, Germany shone more light on how 1,8-cineole helps conditions associated with COPD and asthma. Where previously the consensus of opinion was main benefits of the oil came from its ability to reduce and cut through the mucous in the respiratory tract, their study showed that the constituent also worked as a mediator for the inflammatory response. The assertion from the paper was that "recent clinical trials with 1,8-cineole have shown first evidence for the beneficial use of 1,8-cineole as long-term therapy in the prevention of COPD-exacerbations and to improve asthma control."

In 2014, a team of researchers at Pennsylvania University tested the assumption that eucalyptus, sweet orange, lemon and myrtle essential oils were as effective in treating respiratory disorders as traditional medicine had proposed. They found it speeded the cilia beat frequency and thus improved how quickly mucous is cleared from the respiratory tracts.

A Tunisian team did a fascinating study into the comparative effects if eight different strains of eucalyptus to test their efficacy in the struggle against pathogens such as staphyllocucus aureus, H. influenzi and a whole host of other delightfuls you would not want to invite round for tea. Interestingly whilst our usual and most popular *eucalyptus globulus* was effective in reducing the number of pathogens in the petri dish, it was left standing by another strain *Eucalyptus smithii* which performed far more powerfully. Importantly though, it was found that extracts from the globulus fruits were far more effective than treatments with 1,8-cineole alone supporting the holistic medicine approach of avoiding splitting of components.

Incidentally Dorman and Deans (2000), confirmed that antimicrobial activity increased with oils that were rich in aldehydes, ketones and phenols. If you remember back to the notes in *The Complete Guide to Clinical Aromatherapy and the Essential Oils of the Physical Body*, you will recall that the aldehydes are the some of the first parts of the oil to degrade. Given that then, it is important to replace your bottle every 6-12 months to ensure that it retains its power to bust the bugs.

In a 2004 Study, Lu et al. confirmed Eucalyptus globulus also had an anti-inflammatory effect on bronchitis because it calms the secretion of toxins in the tract. 2003 a team from Brazil tested Eucalyptus citriodora and globulus and verified that the oils not only work as anti-inflammatories but also have analgesic affects.

Safety: Generally regarded as safe. Because of high levels of 1,8 cineole, which can cause depression of the central nervous system and breathing difficulties, do not use on children's faces.

Frankincense

Boswellia carteria

This is probably more for patients with asthma really, because of its ability to slow down the breath. I do find it a very helpful inhalant in those early days of an infection and I cannot catch my breath for coughing too. It seems to me it would be an excellent oil for those who have emphysema to try, because of its restorative quality.

The Frankincense family has been found to modulate MMP12, a precursor to the inflammatory response. Calming MMP12, over time, reduces inflammation in the respiratory tract, opening them and making breathing easier.

Safety: Generally regarded as safe.

High probability of oxidation, so do not use old oils.

Ginger

Zingiber offinale

Proven to be a bronchodilator (opens the airways). Also, useful for reducing temperature in a fever. As always, with my zingy friend, I shall point out that ginger is useful for any condition where the patient is dealing with moisture. So, then indicated in chronic bronchitis too.

Safety: Generally regarded as safe.

Mandarin

Citrus reticulata

Now those of you who read much of my work might have a little giggle that I have managed to sneak my personal favourite oil in, Mandarin, again. It's not really nepotism I promise, because not only does it support the adrenals (which become exhausted after extended use of steroid treatments) but it also has been found to have a direct effect on the scarring of the lungs. An article in 2012 Journal of Chinese Integrative Medicine detailed how *Citrus reticulata* seemed to balance the rate of oxidative stress and down regulate the production of collagen and fibrosis, thus reducing scarring. Just in case it is not obvious: the larger the amount of scarring in the airways, the smaller the space for airflow, making it harder and harder to breathe.

I use this with frankincense and myrrh in a lotion that I rub onto my chest, just below the sternum, every day.

Safety: Generally regarded as safe

Myrtle

Myrtus communis

Proven in 2013, to be a bronchodilator. In 2014 to improve cilia beat frequency and 2015, that it regulates nitric oxide production. Myrtle does contain 1,8 cineole, but is moderate concentrations of typically around 29%. For this reason, this is the oil I use for children's coughs. It is a very safe and gentle oil.

Safety: Generally regarded as safe. Do not use with diabetes medication as there are possible carciniogenic results. Use maximum dilution of 1.9%

Niaouli

Maleleuca quinquinervia

Excellent for disease control, because it kicks the immune system up a gear.

Safety: Generally regarded as safe. Do not use on children's faces as it contains high levels of 1,8 cineole which can depress the central nervous system and cause respiratory complaints.

Oregano

Origanum vulgare

Oregano, or more specifically its active constituent carvacrol increases immunity and fights infection by bringing about cell death of cytokines. This would not necessarily help bronchitis alone, since 2013 trial on patients with colorectal cancer proved oregano helps build immunity but has no system to reduce inflammation. So, only use oregano in cases of flare ups of infection and then skip it the rest of the time. Use other oils to reduce inflammation

Safety: Safety: Generally regarded as safe.

However Tisserand and Young also lists hazards to be aware of:

"Drug interaction; inhibits blood clotting; embryotoxicity; skin irritation (low risk); mucous membrane irritation (moderate risk). Contraindications (all routes): Pregnancy, breastfeeding. Cautions (dermal): Hypersensitive, diseased or damaged skin, children under two years of age. Cautions: anticoagulant medication, major surgery, peptic ulcer,

haemophilia, other bleeding disorders. Maximum dermal use level: 1.1%"

Peppermint

Mentha piperita

Relaxes the airways and also reduces temperature. Peppermint is an extremely stimulating oil. If you use this before bed, you better get used to watching MTV till dawn. Only use in the mornings, but it has a much more pleasant scent than most of these oils so that's a bonus!

Safety: Generally regarded as safe. Not suitable for use in pregnancy. Do not exceed 3% dosage. It is neurotoxic sois contraindicated in cases of epilepsy and patients prone to psychosis, for them reduce to $1/15^{th}$ of drop in a blend. (See homeopathic dose in The Complete Guide to Clinical Aromatherapy.)

Ravensara

Ravensara aromatica

I can find no clinical evidence to support this but it is my go-to oil as soon as I feel an infection coming on. It is antispasmodic to the respiratory tract, expectorant and antiviral. Ravensara, alongside mandarin, is my BFF.

Please be aware of the labelling on your bottle, as two similar oils are confused even by vendors. Ravensara should be labelled *Ravensara aromatic.* If you notice labelling of *Cinnamonum comphora,* this is actually a different oil ravintsara. Ravintsara potentially maybe more useful to you since it has a high level of 1,8 cineole making it extremely beneficial in cases of respiratory problems, but it is a sharper, less benign oil, and I certainly would not want it used on children.

The main constituent in ravensara is limonene meaning it will oxidise very quickly. Ensure you buy small enough bottles to use quickly and often.

Safety: Generally regarded as safe.

Spearmint

Mentha spicata

In 2008 Zhejiang University showed that spearmint had a protective effect on the lung tissues with rats with COPD. It was shown to reduce inflammation and alter oxidation of the tissues. Although gentler than peppermint, still don't tempt the insomnia fairy by using in the evenings.

It's also interesting to see what mum (Jill Bruce) wrote in her book *The Garden of Eden*

"Physical

Feels like thyme, it is very modest, has an affinity with little girls growing up, first periods etc. It can combat the terrible embarrassment of teenage years, help in child abuse cases.

Mental

Helps the transition of things, especially embarrassing or maybe scandalous times. It allows modesty and dignity."

Are we secretly back to treating Adverse Childhood Experiences / trauma again here, I wonder? Dunno...who knows how those clever plants work!

Safety: Generally regarded as safe. Very low risk of skin sensitisation. Tisserand and Young suggest not to use in dilutions of more than 1.7%

Tagetes

Tagetes minuta

My, my, we are racking up the number of frowned upon/hazardous oils here aren't we! I love this beautiful French marigold, but since there have been reports of it causing skin reactions it seems to have dropped out of popularity a bit. It is not an oil I ever worry about using, I have to say.

I'll just copy and paste the conclusion from a 2014 trial in Shiraz, Iran

"T. minuta essential oil has radical scavenging and anti-inflammatory activities and could potentially be used as a safe effective source of natural anti-oxidants in therapy against oxidative damage and stress associated with some inflammatory conditions."

In a trial a month earlier it was described as having "*exhibited high activity against methicillin-resistant Staphylococcus aureus (MRSA)*"

Safety: Can cause photosensitisation and also skin irritation. Is thought to be potentially carcinogenic and inhibits blood clotting. Should not be used in concentrations of more than 0.01%

Thyme

Thymus vulgare

We have already seen it reduces pathogens in the air.

There are many trials confirming that acute bronchitis is helped with a syrup of thyme and ivy. Whilst there is no essential oil of ivy, I can attest to the healing affects of a tincture from A Vogel. (I don't know enough about ivy to give you a recipe to make your own. Sorry!)

It is also anti-inflammatory and anti-microbial as well as being a pulmonary disinfectant. I am a big fan of thyme; it can do a lot of things very well. It is a potent and diverse oil. I expect it to whisper many more in the labs over the next couple of years.

Safety: Moderate dermal irritant so do not use on sensitive or damaged skins and best to avoid use on young children. May inhibit blood clotting. Not suitable for use in pregnancy.

Wintergreen
Gaultheria Procumbens

Because wintergreen is mentioned in the supporting evidence clinical trial in the children's hospital I thought I would cover it here. Certainly there is plenty of data supporting the anti-inflammatory effects of its constituent methyl salicylate, but nothing to suggest it particularly for respiratory complaints. I can however attest to its painkilling abilities and how fast it will clean out the sinuses. There are however better oils listed through the book. Keep wintergreen for your bad knees!

Safety: Hazards: Drug interaction; inhibits blood clotting; toxicity; high doses cause birth defects.

Contraindications (all routes): Anticoagulant medication, major surgery, haemophilia, other bleeding disorders

Pregnancy, breastfeeding, children. People with salicylate sensitivity (often applies in ADD/ ADHD). Contraindications Maximum dermal use level: 2.4%. The risks of systemic toxicity are heightened by application onto damaged skin.

Yarrow

Achillea millefolium

My beautiful blue yarrow, how I love thee! It is such a benign and special oil. In 2011, in Pakistan, it was proven to relax and open the airways. In addition to its bronchodilatory effects, they announced proof that it reduces blood pressure and reduces hyperactive cardiovascular activity.

In 2013, its anti-inflammatory affects were identified as down regulating the release of nitric oxide and IL-6, thereby reducing oxidative stress.

It is a powerful antifungal against a whole host of mouldy miscreants, including *aspergillus niger* and *aspergillus fumigatus*

Safety: In strong dilutions is neurotoxic and so should not be used in cases of epilepsy or possible psychosis.

Carrier oils

In a study into the affects of essential oils and carriers, sesame and peanut/groundnut oils both improved *nasal* cilia beat frequency. Although it is not ground breaking evidence into bronchitis or COPD per se, I think we would be silly to ignore it. (A high five for Ayurvedic medicine who have long used sesame in their nasal cleanses!)

Also for anti-inflammatory effects, I would suggest coconut oil, sea buckthorn (be careful it does not stain you, use only a smidge) borage oils and, of course, evening primrose.

In some ways, this section goes against everything I believe in. Everyone is ill for a different reason, and so in truth no one recipe can treat all ills. There can never be a one size fits all solution, because the number of things affecting the patient are myriad, but perhaps more importantly so are the possible contraindications from treatments. It is for the second reason that I have erred on the side of caution with these recipes.

Please do not take these recipes to be the *be all and end all* of your therapy. There are plenty of clues throughout the book to oils that can help you to get better; be innovative, create beautiful perfumes from them, take incredible baths...become proficient.

On occasion I have added recommendations for carrier oils, which would denote they are to be used as massage oils...but that's only guidance. Use them as evaporator oils, drip them into the bath, adapt and utilise.

Bear in mind too, there is no reason why you can't address several conditions at once. If you want to uplift your mood and open your airways as well as find infection...knock yourself out. Go for it, there are no rules here, only opportunities for health.

Now, importantly there is no safety data in this section, because I intend for you to double check against my book *The*

Complete Guide to Clinical Aromatherapy and The Essential Oils of The Physical Body. The title is long enough to type on its own, let alone to list all the safety data too. There are directions about how create compresses, do massages etc. The book is free, it took me months to create; please use it!

One last thing, my blends are not necessarily synergistically blended either. This is pure idleness on my part. Feel free to mess about with notes to get top, middle and base and potentially the effects will be stronger still. Again there are notes on this is in The Complete Guide, as well as a blending chart. If you need to feel free to download again at http://www.buildyourownreality.com/blending-notes

So, let's start where the doctor starts with the physical healing, then we can peel back more layers.

Physical Healing

Bronchitis Massage Oil

100ml / 4fl oz carrier oil

Eucalyptus x 2

Frankincense x 2

Mandarin x

Myrtle x3

Children's Bronchitis Oil

Use this blend on their feet and backs, not on their chests please. I find it helps to give them a soothing foot massage, taking in the reflex and acupressure point on their feet then put their socks on when they go to bed

100ml Evening Primrose / borage oil

Myrtle x 3 drop

Camomile roman x 1 drop

Eucalyptus x 1 drop

Tea tree x 1 drop

Silver fir x 1 drop

Children's bath

Add 2 drops of myrtle with 1 drop lavender to help them sleep.

Massage Oil / Lotion for Infection

25ml / 1oz Borage Carrier oil

Tea tree x 3 drops

Ravensara x 1 drop

Clove x 1 drop

Cinnamon x 1 drop

Thyme x 1 drop

Open and Relax Airways

100ml / 4fl oz evening primrose oil

Frankincense x 2 drops

Yarrow x 1 drop

Myrtle x 2 drops

Ginger x 1 drop

Inhalant

Whilst I am writing recipes for this, my feelings are: you can't beat sucking the fumes directly from a tea tree bottle. Do not put your lips on the bottle; we are sucking fumes, not oil. Try to gasp the oil into your throat, a couple of gasps is plenty.

The following blends are to be used in a bowl of hot water. Cover your head with a towel to trap the steam. Keep your head far enough away from the bowl on to scald. Try to breathe slowly and deeply to take in the fumes. 2-3 minutes at a time is ample.

Inhalant Blend for Infection

Tea tree x 1 drop

Ravensara x 1 drop

Manuka x 1 drop

Induce Mucous in Acute Bronchitis Dry Cough

Benzoin x 2 drop

Rose x 1 drop

Camomile x 1 drop

Clear sinuses in upper respiratory infection

Lemon x 1 drop

Myrrh x 1 drop

Tea tree x 1 drop

Wound Healing for Emphysema

In a 100g blank ointment / lotion or moisturiser base.

Litsea Cubeba x 1

Lemon grass x 1

Petitgrain x 2

Geranium x 2

Myrrh x3

Quit smoking

I can't imagine essential oils would go very far on their own with this, but I have mixed a blend of oils believed to help with addiction. Black pepper has seen good results on its own. That said, please see the doctor for support and more proven methods to help you quit.

One such method, is hypnotherapy, and as ever I recommend you visit www.buildyourownreality.com/mark-bowden-hypnotherapy/ to check out his quit smoking recordings.

Black pepper x 1 drop

Aniseed x 1 drop

Cypress x 3 drops

Lemon verbena x 2 drops

Cleansing Room Spray

Clean down your environment with cassia to reduce the impact of aspergillus and dust on your lungs. Because it is such a no-nonsense oil, I have tempered its reality check aspects with sunnier and relaxing oils.

Lemon Verbena is believed to remove cigarettes smoke from the environment. Again though, this is no substitute for getting cigarettes out of your house.

Incidentally, I do like my steam cleaner, because it can get to the places other cleaners can't reach! I tried adding the oils to the steamer to see if I could get a fumigation effect. Didn't work! It just seemed to reduce the amount of steam that came out of the gadget. Never mind, spray your oils then blitz with the steamer (or vice versa, I don't suppose it matters!)

PS wear some gloves. Don't get this one on your hands. It will sting.

Lemon verbena x 3 drops

Cassia x 2 drops

Thyme x 2 drops

Patchouli x 6 drops

Oils for the Emotions

Relaxation in the bath

Lavender x 2 drops

Marjoram x 1 drops

Geranium x 2 drops

Confidence and independence

In a 100 ml lotion

Frankincense x 5 drops

Coriander x 2 drops

Spearmint x 2 drops

Trust
In a 25 ml (1oz) lotion

Geranium x 2 drops

Cypress x 1 drops

Ylang Ylang x 2 drops

Essential oils to lift trauma
100ml rosehip carrier oil

Oakmoss resin x 1 drop

Amber x 1 drop

Rose x 3 drops

Spiritual Adjustments
I suppose really, this is the area that turns the physical breathing dysfunction into the emotional depression we see developing in so many patients.

Dependency on oxygen, the inability to do things that were once so simple, the lack of control over one's own life and future are all feelings that can take control.

So, I have blended oils that allow the mind the let these things go, and enjoy life for what it is

In a diffuser

Bergamot x 3 drops

Thyme x 1 drops

Cardamom x 3 drops

Peripheral Problems Connected with COPD

Insomnia
100ml / 40z lotion, in a diffuser or in the bath. Full on attack!

Lavender x 3 drops

Marjoram x 1 drops

Valerian x 3 drops

Yarrow x 2 drops

Neck and Shoulder Massage Oil
100ml 40z Coconut oil

10ml sea buckthorn

Lavender x 3 drops

Juniper x 2 drops

Black pepper x 1 drop

Swollen Ankles

Compresses, footbaths, lotions

Geranium x 2 drops

Cypress x 2 drops

Fennel x 1 drop

To Combat Weight Loss and Loss of Appetite

100 ml lotion

Tarragon x 2 drops

Basil x 2 drops

Angelica x 4 drops

Fatigue

100 ml 4 oz lotion

Mandarin x 2 drops

Rosemary x 1 drop

Bergamot x 4 drops

Aromapendants

One last treat. It is a *how- to* rather than a recipe. I have a new hobby....making aromatic jewellery. As many of you will know I adore cake decorating and so have loads of little cutters for flowers and leaves. I have been using these to cut out shapes to make beautiful respiratory necklaces. For an easier option, why not just cut yourself a simple disc and stamp a design on.

Honestly, these are ace!

Visit your local craft shop and treat yourself to some clay.

Roll and cut out shapes, or make small beads.

Use a large needle or punch to make a hole large enough to thread your string or thong through

Leave to dry

The clay then becomes very porous and will hold your essential oils

Put one drop of oil on each bead or shape. Just in case of staining, do the back of each one.

(I like to "code" mine: one type of leaf gets eucalyptus, another gets ravensara etc This way if I have created a blend 4 x euc, 4 x lav, 2 x ravensara, it is easy to work how many beads I need of each) Paint them up if you like! Thread on and wear your medicine in style!!!

Conclusion

Wow, what an adventure. Putting this book together has had me marvelling every step of the way. Not least because my late step father Michael Cook was a devil for using hazardous oils. When I inherited his oils box when he died, I described it as a weapon of mass destruction. He had always maintained that they were the best way to treat inflammation, and so far this research leads me to suspect we might find he may have been right. We'll see.

For you of course, that journey is just beginning. Know that I am here with you every step of the way. I spend an unhealthy amount of time looking at facbook.com/TheSecretHealerWrites and you can always send me questions there if you feel you need extra aromatherapy support. Do remember, please to wipe your nose and wash your hands before you turn up !

Kendall-Tacketts work has highlighted to me the need for a book that fills in the gaps of how sleep and relaxation affects our health, and so I am off to research that next. I aim to release that at the end of Feb 2015, but the month might be a bit short for that...! Don't forget to click follow on my author page on Amazon if you want an alert.

In the meantime, try to remember what I said

Relax...take a chill pill....breathe....

I hope you have found the research interesting and helpful. A big thank you to those of you who have posted reviews on my other books, they are extremely helpful to me, and I do enjoy reading your comments. Please can I ask you all to try to find a moment to comment on this one, too.

Review and buy! Bye !

Acknowledgements

Thank you so much to John Stoddart for your review on Google Play that made me giggle and decide to seize the spelling issue with both hands.

The pyramid of the Adverse Childhood Experiences is reproduced with thanks for the Wikemedia Commons community. The beautiful opening quote is reproduced from goodreads.com.

The artwork on the cover and the downloads are magically created by the wonderful Robert Elsmore of Robert Elsmore Images.

Thanks to every one of you in the facbook, linked in, twitter and Amazon communities for your endless support and love, especially to Jeanne, who has become my official (and much adored) stalker. She has earned her esteemed title by sharing absolutely everything I say on her networks. Here's to you Jeanne; your fifteen minutes of fame xxx

About the Author

Elizabeth Ashley qualified as an aromatherapist in 1993, and then passed her Advanced Aromatherapy Diploma in 1994. She has been practicing aromatherapy for almost 21 years.

In 1999, she fell into a whole new career in the aggressive commercial sector of recruitment consultancy. There she discovered her father's second hand car salesman genes had passed along and found she had quite a gift of the gab! More than that, she discovered she could sell...and then some.

In 2008, Elizabeth fell ill during pregnancy with a blood clot in her lungs. The pulmonary embolism prevented her from working and she started to write. Very quickly she gained her first contract as a ghost writer...a recipe book for cheese cakes!

In 2010 she was published professionally for her work on Galbanum oil in the Aromatherapy Thymes, journal of the International Federation of Aromatherapists, and on Tuberose oil by the New Zealand Register of Holistic Therapist.

In 2011 she was seconded on a consultative basis to Walsall Independent Treatment Centre, designed to be a rainbow bridge between traditional and complementary medicines. There she became aware of the rumblings of change in healthcare. Her book *Sales Strategies for Gentle Souls* explains the connotations of this.

Many of her books are aimed at helping qualified aromatherapists to expand their healing repertoire and build their businesses. She also writes for people who have an interest in essential oils and want to learn how to heal. Her in depth essential oil profiles chart the healing properties of plants from the most arcane depths of historic folklore up to the scientific lab trials of today.

In 2014 she ranks in the top 50 contract writers on the freelancer marketplace Elance.com. She is the ghost writer of seven number one Amazon best sellers in the natural healing category. She lives in Shropshire with her husband and youngest son, kept company by their cat, the budgie and many shoals of tropical fish! Her elder son and daughter attend University and make her prouder than anything ever could.

Elizabeth Ashley is possibly one of the most published aromatherapy writers you have never heard of! By 2015, all of that will have changed. Elizabeth Ashley is *The Secret Healer*.

Other books in The Secret Healer Series

Book 1 - The Complete Guide to

Clinical Aromatherapy & Essential Oils for the Physical Body

Essentially...essential oils for beginners, talented novices and intermediate aromatherapists

Let me ask you, why do you want a book on aromatherapy?

Do you want to learn how to care for your family naturally?

Perhaps you have a franchise selling essential oils and want to know more about what they can do?

Maybe you love the delicious scents and want understand how these beautiful things come to heal.

I wonder if you have started to learn and now want to discover how to build on your knowledge.

Whatever you are looking for this book has something for you.

- Details of how to treat over 60 conditions with essential oils
- Profiles of over 100 natural plant essences and their safety data
- Descriptions of 15 carrier oils and their applications not only for massage but also adding to creams and lotions.

- Comprehensive data of how the chemistry of an oil will affect its actions
- In depth insights into how professional aromatherapists blend...including their 13 favourite recipes from their practices.

Including....

- Sensuous aromatherapy blends by a qualified sex therapist
- Two blends for labour by the midwife running an aromatherapy program on an NHS maternity ward
- A blend for depression by a qualified mental health

PLUS....

10 bonus essential oil monographs and a complementary hypnotherapy relaxation download.

Discount vouchers of treatments courses and products by participating therapists.

AND.... for those of you who would like to contribute, there is a chance to make a donation to cancer research too.

This is my gift to you.

<u>Download for FREE - From 30.11.14</u>

Book 2 Essential Oils for Mind Body Spirit

The Holistic Medicine of Clinical Aromatherapy

Healing the skin, easing the tummy ache or getting someone to sleep is easy with essential oils. Anyone can do it. The joy of healing, though, comes from peeling back the layers of the disease, almost like a detective to find out exactly what caused it in the first place.

Consider this book to be lesson 2 in The Secret Healer Series.

You have mastered which oil to use for what and why...this book takes you step by step though the ancient healing mechanisms of the aura, the chakras and meridians but also explores how that ties in with the latest scientific discoveries into how the emotions affect our health. Using Candace Pert's remarkable "Molecules of Emotion" research, The Secret Healer shows you *where* to look for healing links and *why*.

- Uncover how a certain recurrent negative emotion can be the trigger to make you ill?
- Understand internal processes that mean that psychology, neurology and immunology are quintessentially, and inextricably linked.
- Learn how to use essential oils control your emotions and in turn bring about a far greater standard of wellness.

- Discover mindblowing research that shows the emotions we experience are actually the sensations of neuropeptides triggering our organs to do their jobs
- Reflect on the wonder of Chinese medicine and ancient healing being completely accurate in their healing mechanisms for thousands of years...now that science proves it to be so.

Essential Oils for The Mind Body Spirit couples ancient wisdom with cutting edge science. This is the knowledge the drug companies hope you never find out and our doctors pray we all will.

A short write up, for a book that will change your life. I promise you, when you read the latest findings of psychoimmunolgy, you will never waster another day on being angry again.

<u>Book 3 The Essential Oil Liver Cleanse</u>

The Professional Aromatherapist's Liver Detox

We are warned of the threats of heart attacks, strokes and cancer, especially if we are overweight.

What is kept quieter is doctors have established a link between toxicity in the liver and metabolic syndrome, the condition that leads to many of these conditions. What's more non fatty liver disease is known to underlie many other conditions such as ezcema, allergies and headaches.

The scandal is just how many of our livers are struggling under the strain of over processed foods, pharmaceutical debris and actually even our own bad tempers!

This book explains:

- The importance of the liver and its functions
- How it becomes dysfunctional and how to interpret warning signposts
- How to cleanse and nourish using not just essential oils, but also vitamins and minerals and diet.
- The strange correlation between how our emotions translate negativity into disease.
- How to implement other therapies such as chiropractic, acupressure and counselling and how to secure fantastic referrals.

This book is best used in tandem with The Professional Stress Solution to benefit from the complementary healing. Use Sales Strategies for Gentle Souls to create a marketing plan to use your new found knowledge to smash your competition out of the water!!!

Book 4 The Professional Stress Solution

Essential Oils and Holistic Health Stress Management Techniques for The Professional Aromatherapist

Stress is pandemic in our society.

Scientists agree it plays a quintessential role in how likely it is we will suffer from chronic and possibly fatal illnesses in the future. Risk factors of metabolic syndrome, diabetes, stroke and heart disease are increased through stress.

The daft thing is....aromatherapy can do amazing things to ease it, and potentially aromatherapists could take a massive workload away from the doctor's surgeries.

- Discover the hormonal changes and peptide triggers that change a person's health and mental state.
- Learn how it affects the liver, adrenals and pituitary gland.
- Uncover the strange phenomenon of Yin disease
- Build a better foundation of care, but also a knowledge base that means you can sell your treatments more effectively.
- Improve your healing skills set
- Supercharge your referrals potential from other complementary therapists and orthodox medicine alike.

Includes free bonus material of

- Chiropractic chart of misalignments and potential organic disturbance
- Chart of the meridians and suggested acupressure points to detox the organs more quickly
- Detailed information about how to improve the patients condition with vitamin and minerals therapy
- In depth dietary advice
- Free hypnotherapy relaxation download

Essential Oils are The Off Switch for stress. The *Professional Stress Solution* is the ON SWITCH for your aromatherapy business.

Book 5 The Aromatherapy Eczema Treatment

Healing Eczema, Itchy Skin Rashes and Atopic Dermatitis with Essential Oils and Holistic Medicine

Most people appreciate that the itching and redness of eczema can be used using essential oils, but what if I told you they were capable of so much more?

Imagine if, as a therapist, you were able to pinpoint the emotions that set off these flares? Can you visualise what it would mean to your patient if you were able to isolate the very protagonist causing the eczema breakout and alleviate their pain completely?

Well now you can.

This book teaches you:

- How to isolate the emotions causing the emotional cycle of pain
- The likely food triggers for your patient and the tools to identify the exact times they will detonate a reaction
- The familial traits and links that lead to atopic eczema
- How these links connect with the liver and in turn how to cleanse the liver toxicity
- Vitamins and minerals to cleanse and nourish the system

The book contains very real that will not only transform the way you treat clients, but will skyrocket your clinic's takings.

I recommend reading this book in tandem with *The Professional Stress Solution* and the *Essential Oil Liver Cleanse* to fully understand the cycles and processes of treatment. Add to it *Sales Strategies for Gentle Souls* and your business will stand on an entirely new footing.

Why not save yourself 1/3

And treat yourself to the set?

The full and comprehensive course into how to heal eczema

with aromatherapy and essential oils **$9.99 / £5.99**

Sales Strategies for Gentle Souls

Targeted Sales Training for Professional Aromatherapists

Wonderful things are happening in complementary therapy. Very gifted people are churning out fantastic research and results. The internet is full of what essential oils can do. But when a gentle soul emerges from their relaxing haze of their aromatherapy class room, how do they harness the buzz of energy around them for their craft?

From 1999-2008 I worked in one of the most aggressive commercial environments there is. My role as a recruitment consultant was 80% cold calling in an extremely saturated sales arena. Despite my own gentle soul, I found ways not only to compete, but to excel.

- Learn how to pinpoint the best customers for your practice
- Cost your treatments to ensure every treatment is profitable for both you and your customer
- Discover how to make every conversation into a potential sale lead without becoming a complete and utter pain in the a*s!
- Uncover the reasons why you are not closing sales so you never have to make the same mistakes again
- Create a growth environment where you plan success and always find yourself stepping into it

If you are working with essential oils, and you want to make a good living for it, then you need to learn to sell. What's more, if you are going to say "selling doesn't work on my customers"....then you have simply been taught to do it wrongly.

My dream is to see aromatherapy at the forefront of medicine. I need an army of gifted healers to achieve that. Consider yourself to be my newest recruit and I am going to drill you till you are the slickest, subtlest and most effective marketeer there is. You have the knowledge to make people better, now let me give you the business prowess to heal even more people than you have ever done before.

The Secret Healer has stress in her sights and she's about to make a killing. Listen carefully...she has much to tell you. £1.99 / $2.99

Buy now

www.thesecrethealer.co.uk

www.buildyourownreality.com

In 2015, Elizabeth Ashley will also publish a new essential oil profile on Amazon each week. See her author profile on Amazon for the latest releases.

Works Cited

Abu-Darwish MS1, C. C.-b. (2013, 10 09). *Essential oil of common sage (Salvia officinalis L.) from Jordan: assessment of safety in mammalian cells and its antifungal and anti-inflammatory potential.* Retrieved 01 08, 2015, from Pubmed: http://www.ncbi.nlm.nih.gov/pubmed/24224168

Alvarez MV1, O.-R. L.-P.-M.-G.-A.-Z. (2014, 12 14). *Oregano essential oil-pectin edible films as anti-quorum sensing and food antimicrobial agents.* Retrieved 01 22, 2015, from Pubmed: http://www.ncbi.nlm.nih.gov/pubmed/25566215

Ashley, E. (2014). *The Complete Guide To Clinical Aromatherapy and The Essential Oils of The Physical Body.* Build Your Own Reality.

Ashley, E. (2014). *The Essential Oils of The Mind Body Spirit.* Build Your Own Reality.

Ashley, E. (2014). *The Professional Stress Solution* . Build Your Own Reality.

Bilcu M1, G. A. (2014, 11 04). *Efficiency of vanilla, patchouli and ylang ylang essential oils stabilized by iron oxide@C14 nanostructures against bacterial adherence and biofilms formed by Staphylococcus aureus and Klebsiella pneumoniae clinical strains.* Retrieved 01 22, 2015, from Pubmed: http://www.ncbi.nlm.nih.gov/pubmed/25375335

Bimczok D1, R. H. (2008, 04 22). *Influence of carvacrol on proliferation and survival of porcine lymphocytes and intestinal epithelial cells in vitro.* Retrieved 01 22, 2015, from Pubmed: http://www.ncbi.nlm.nih.gov/pubmed/18267355

Bouaziz M1, Y. T. (2009, 11). *Disinfectant properties of essential oils from Salvia officinalis L. cultivated in Tunisia.*

Retrieved 01 08, 2015, from Pubmed: http://www.ncbi.nlm.nih.gov/pubmed/19682532

Bouzabata A1, C. C. (2015, 01). *Myrtus communis L. as source of a bioactive and safe essential oil.* Retrieved 01 23, 2015, from Pubmed: http://www.ncbi.nlm.nih.gov/pubmed/25446467

Bruce, J. (1994). Advanced Diploma of Aromatherapy. *Jill Bruce School of Aromatherapy* .

Bruce, J. (1993). Diploma Course of Aromatherapy. *Jill Bruce School of Aromatherapy* .

Bruce, J. (2014). *The Aura.* Build Your Own Reality.

Bruce, J. (1993). *The Garden of Eden* . Walsall: Magdalena Press.

Bruce, J. (1994). *The Garden of Eden* . Magdelena Press.

Chen H1, Y. Y. (2014, 06 14). *Comparison of compositions and antimicrobial activities of essential oils from chemically stimulated agarwood, wild agarwood and healthy Aquilaria sinensis (Lour.) gilg trees.* Retrieved 01 22, 2015, from Pubmed: http://www.ncbi.nlm.nih.gov/pubmed/21677602

Chiropractic America. (n.d.). *Chronic Bronchitis.* Retrieved 21 2015, 2015, from Your Spine.com: http://www.yourspine.com/Chiropractor/Chronic+Conditions/Bronchitis.aspx

Chou ST1, P. H. (2013, 06 24). *Achillea millefolium L. Essential Oil Inhibits LPS-Induced Oxidative Stress and Nitric Oxide Production in RAW 264.7 Macrophages.* Retrieved 01 26, 2015, from Pubmed: http://www.ncbi.nlm.nih.gov/pubmed/23797659

Claudio Cermelli, A. F. (2007, 08 27). *The effects of Eucalyptus oil on respiratory bacteria and viruses*. Retrieved 01 22, 2015, from Current Microbioloigy: http://link.springer.com/article/10.1007%2Fs00284-007-9045-0#page-1

Cohen HA1, R. J. (2012, 09). *Effect of honey on nocturnal cough and sleep quality: a double-blind, randomized, placebo-controlled study*. Retrieved 01 23, 2015, from Pubmed: http://www.ncbi.nlm.nih.gov/pubmed/22869830

Davis, P. (1993). *Aromatherapy and A-Z*. Saffron Waldron, Essex: C W Daniel Company.

Day, B. J. (2008, 02). *Antioxidants as Potential Therapeutics for Lung Fibrosis*. Retrieved 01 25, 2015, from Pubmed: http://www.ncbi.nlm.nih.gov/pmc/articles/PMC2660674/

de Sousa AA1, S. P. (2010, 06 20). *Antispasmodic effect of Mentha piperita essential oil on tracheal smooth muscle of rats*. Retrieved 01 22, 2015, from Pubmed: http://www.ncbi.nlm.nih.gov/pubmed/20488237

Dibazar SP1, F. S. (2014, 05 30). *Immunomodulatory effects of clove (Syzygium aromaticum) constituents on macrophages: In vitro evaluations of aqueous and ethanolic components*. Retrieved 01 22, 2015, from Pubmed: http://www.ncbi.nlm.nih.gov/pubmed/24873744

European Molecular Biology Laboratory. (2003, 08 03). *Scientists open doors to diagnosis of emphysema*. Retrieved 01 22, 2015, from Phys.org: http://phys.org/news168510886.html

Fabio A1, C. C. (2007, 04 04). *Screening of the antibacterial effects of a variety of essential oils on microorganisms responsible for respiratory infections*. Retrieved 01 22, 2015,

from Pubmed:
http://www.ncbi.nlm.nih.gov/pubmed/17326042

Falconieri D1, P. A. (2011, 10 06). *Chemical composition and biological activity of the volatile extracts of Achillea millefolium*. Retrieved 01 026, 2015, from Pubmed:
http://www.ncbi.nlm.nih.gov/pubmed/22164800

Hari K. Koul, M. P. (2013). *Role of p38 MAP Kinase Signal Transduction in Solid Tumors*. Retrieved 01 23, 2015, from Genes Cancer:
http://www.ncbi.nlm.nih.gov/pmc/articles/PMC3863344/

Hässig A1, L. W. (2000). *Bronchial asthma: information on phytotherapy with essential fatty acids. Interactions between essential fatty acids and steroid hormones*. Retrieved 01 23, 2015, from Pubmed:
http://www.ncbi.nlm.nih.gov/pubmed/10790728

Increases In Exhaled Nitric Oxide After Acute stress: Association With Measures of Negative Affect And Depressive Mood. (2014, 12). Retrieved 01 13, 2015, from Journal of Psychosomatic Medicine:
http://journals.lww.com/psychosomaticmedicine/Abstract/2014/11000/Increases_in_Exhaled_Nitric_Oxide_After_Acute.8.aspx

Inouye S1, T. T. (2001, 05). *Antibacterial activity of essential oils and their major constituents against respiratory tract pathogens by gaseous contact*. Retrieved 01 22, 2015, from Pubmed: http://www.ncbi.nlm.nih.gov/pubmed/11328766

Jann-Yuan Wang, 1. P.-R.-T.-N.-C.-T. (2000). *Recurrent Infections and Chronic Colonization by an Escherichia coli Clone in the Respiratory Tract of a Patient with Severe Cystic Bronchiectasis*. Retrieved 08 01, 2015, from Journal of clinical

microbiology:
http://www.ncbi.nlm.nih.gov/pmc/articles/PMC87025/

Karimian P1, K. G. (2014, 03 04). *Anti-oxidative and anti-inflammatory effects of Tagetes minuta essential oil in activated macrophages.* Retrieved 01 2015, 2015, from Pubmed: http://www.ncbi.nlm.nih.gov/pubmed/25182441

Karimian P1, K. G. (2014, 03). *Anti-oxidative and anti-inflammatory effects of Tagetes minuta essential oil in activated macrophages.* Retrieved 01 26, 2015, from Pubmed: http://www.ncbi.nlm.nih.gov/pubmed/25182441

Kedia A1, P. B. (2014, 01 03). *Antifungal and antiaflatoxigenic properties of Cuminum cyminum (L.) seed essential oil and its efficacy as a preservative in stored commodities.* Retrieved 01 08, 2015, from Pubmed: http://www.ncbi.nlm.nih.gov/pubmed/24211773

Kent, N. (2012). *Glossary of Symptoms.* Retrieved 01 26, 2015, from My Holistic Healing.com: http://www.my-holistic-healing.com/mind-body-connection-kidneys.html

Kilina AV, K. M. (2011). *[The efficacy of the application of essential oils for the prevention of acute respiratory diseases in organized groups of children].* Retrieved 01 29, 2015, from Medi.ru: http://www.medi.ru/doc/a601005.htm

Kim HK1, Y. Y. (2008, 01). *Fumigant toxicity of cassia bark and cassia and cinnamon oil compounds to Dermatophagoides farinae and Dermatophagoides pteronyssinus (Acari: Pyroglyphidae).* Retrieved 01 22, 2015, from Pubmed:
http://www.ncbi.nlm.nih.gov/pubmed/18247142

Kitic D1, P. D. (2013). *The role of essential oils and the biological detoxification in the prevention of aflatoxin borne diseases*. Retrieved 01 08, 2015, from Pubmed: http://www.ncbi.nlm.nih.gov/pubmed/24083787

Kocevski D1, D. M. (2013, 05). *Antifungal effect of Allium tuberosum, Cinnamomum cassia, and Pogostemon cablin essential oils and their components against population of Aspergillus species*. Retrieved 01 22, 2015, from pUBMED: http://www.ncbi.nlm.nih.gov/pubmed/23647469

Lai Y1, D. D. (2014, May 28). *In vitro studies of a distillate of rectified essential oils on sinonasal components of mucociliary clearance*. Retrieved 01 18, 20147, from Pubmed: http://www.ncbi.nlm.nih.gov/pubmed/24980236

Lu XQ1, T. F. (2004). *Effect of Eucalyptus globulus oil on lipopolysaccharide-induced chronic bronchitis and mucin hypersecretion in rats*. Retrieved 01 20, 2015, from Pubmed: http://www.ncbi.nlm.nih.gov/pubmed/15719688

Mangprayool T1, K. S. (2013, 09). *Participation of citral in the bronchodilatory effect of ginger oil and possible mechanism of action*. Retrieved 01 22, 2015, from pUBMED: http://www.ncbi.nlm.nih.gov/pubmed/23685048

Materia Aromatica. (2015). *Ravintsara versus Ravensara*. Retrieved 01 23, 2015, from Materia aromatica.com: http://materiaaromatica.com/Default.aspx?go=Article&ArticleID=187

Motiejūnaite O1, P. D. (2004). *Fungicidal properties of Pinus sylvestris L. for improvement of air quality*. Retrieved 01 08, 2015, from Pubmed: http://www.ncbi.nlm.nih.gov/pubmed/15300001

Nam SY1, C. M. (2008). *Essential oil of niaouli preferentially potentiates antigen-specific cellular immunity and cytokine production by macrophages*. Retrieved 01 22, 2015, from Pubmed: http://www.ncbi.nlm.nih.gov/pubmed/18668393

Nam SY1, C. M. (2008). *Essential oil of niaouli preferentially potentiates antigen-specific cellular immunity and cytokine production by macrophages*. Retrieved 01 23, 2015, from Pubmed: http://www.ncbi.nlm.nih.gov/pubmed/18668393

Neher A1, G. M. (2008, 03 22). *Influence of essential and fatty oils on ciliary beat frequency of human nasal epithelial cells*. Retrieved 01 22, 2015, from Pubmed: http://www.ncbi.nlm.nih.gov/pubmed/18416967

Neher A1, G. M. (2008, 03). *Influence of essential and fatty oils on ciliary beat frequency of human nasal epithelial cells*. Retrieved 01 26, 2015, from Pubmed: http://www.ncbi.nlm.nih.gov/pubmed/18416967

Pannee C1, C. I. (2014, 10 14). *Antiinflammatory effects of essential oil from the leaves of Cinnamomum cassia and cinnamaldehyde on lipopolysaccharide-stimulated J774A.1 cells*. Retrieved 01 22, 2015, from Pubmed: http://www.ncbi.nlm.nih.gov/pubmed/25364694

Phd, C. P. (2012). *Molecules Of Emotion: Why You Feel The Way You Feel* . Simon & Schuster UK. Kindle Edition.

Poul Suadicani, 1. H. (2011, 06 27). *High Salt Intake and Risk of Chronic Bronchitis: The Copenhagen Male Study—A 10-Year Followup*. Retrieved 01 21, 2015, from Hindawi.com: http://www.hindawi.com/journals/isrn/2011/257979/

Powell, R. (n.d.). *Interactive Spine- Nerve Impingement*. Retrieved 01 21, 2015, from Roger Powell Chiropractic: http://www.chirokzn.co.za/i-spine_T1-T4.html

Ravi AK, K. S. (2014, 09 14). *Increased levels of soluble interleukin-6 receptor and CCL3 in COPD sputum*. Retrieved 01 13, 2015, from Pubmed: http://www.ncbi.nlm.nih.gov/pubmed/25183374

Roy S1, K. S. (2006, 04 08). *Regulation of vascular responses to inflammation: inducible matrix metalloproteinase-3 expression in human microvascular endothelial cells is sensitive to antiinflammatory Boswellia*. Retrieved 01 23, 2015, from Pubmed: http://www.ncbi.nlm.nih.gov/pubmed/?term=MmP12+boswellia

Sanderson, P. D. (2006). *Ciliary Beat Frequency Is Maintained at a Maximal Rate in the Small Airways of Mouse Lung Slices*. Retrieved 01 22, 2015, from ATS Journals: http://www.atsjournals.org/doi/full/10.1165/rcmb.2005-0417OC#.VMEXX8msXUJ

Seca AM1, G. A. (2011, 06 04). *The genus Inula and their metabolites: from ethnopharmacological to medicinal uses*. Retrieved 01 23, 2015, from Pubmed: http://www.ncbi.nlm.nih.gov/pubmed/24754913

Shapiro, D. (2007). *Your body speaks your mind*. Piatkus.

Shirazi MT1, G. H. (2014, 03 02). *Chemical composition, antioxidant, antimicrobial and cytotoxic activities of Tagetes minuta and Ocimum basilicum essential oils*. Retrieved 01 08, 2015, from Pubmed: http://www.ncbi.nlm.nih.gov/pubmed/24804073

Sivamani P, S. G. (2012). *Comparative molecular docking analysis of essential oil constituents as elastase inhibitors*. Retrieved 01 23, 2015, from Pubmed: http://www.ncbi.nlm.nih.gov/pubmed/22715299

Suttie, E. (Unknown). *Dealing with Grief; A TCM perspective*. Retrieved 01 206, 2015, from Chinese Medicine Living: http://www.chinesemedicineliving.com/blog/philosophy/the-emotions/grief-the-lungs/

Tisserand, R., & Young, R. (.-1.-0. (2013). Agarwood. In *Essential Oil Safety: A Guide for Health Care Professionals* (pp. Kindle Locations 12825-12826)). Elsevier Health Sciences UK. Kindle Edition.

Tisserand, R., & Young, R. (.-1.-0. Anise. In *Essential Oil Safety: A Guide for Health Care Professionals* (pp. Kindle Locations 13160-13163). Elsevier Health Sciences UK. Kindle Edition. .

Tisserand, R., & Young, R. (.-1.-0. (2013). Benzoin. In R. Y. Robert Tisserand, *Essential Oil Safety: A Guide for Health Care Professionals* (pp. Kindle Locations 13983-13984). Elsevier Health Sciences UK. Kindle Edition.

Tisserand, R., & Young, R. (.-1.-0. Bergamot. In *Essential Oil Safety: A Guide for Health Care Professionals* (pp. Kindle Locations 14040-14043). Elsevier Health Sciences UK. Kindle Edition. .

(2013). Cinnamon Leaf. In R. Tisserand, & R. Young, *Essential Oil Safety: A Guide for Health Care Professionals* (pp. Kindle Locations 16175-16187). Elsevier Health Sciences UK. Kindle Edition. .

(2013). Clove Bud. In R. Tisserand, & R. Young, *Essential Oil Safety: A Guide for Health Care Professionals* (pp. Kindle Locations 16478-16479). Elsevier Health Sciences UK. Kindle Edition.

U.R. JUERGENS*, U. S. (2002). *Anti-in£ammatory activity of1.8 -cineol (eucalyptol) in bronchial asthma: a double-blind* *placebo-controlled trial.* Retrieved 01 18, 2015, from Aromamd.net: http://www.aromamd.net/edu_asthma.pdf

UR1., J. (2014, 12 01). *Anti-inflammatory Properties of the Monoterpene 1.8-cineole: Current Evidence for Co-medication in Inflammatory Airway Diseases.* Retrieved 01 18, 2015, from Pubmed: http://www.ncbi.nlm.nih.gov/pubmed/24831245

UR1., J. (2014, 12). *Anti-inflammatory Properties of the Monoterpene 1.8-cineole: Current Evidence for Co-medication in Inflammatory Airway Diseases.* Retrieved 01 22, 2015, from Pubmed: http://www.ncbi.nlm.nih.gov/pubmed/24831245

Valnet, D. J. (1996). *The Practice of Aromatherapy.* Saffron Waldron, Essex: C W Daniel Company Ltd.

Vigo E1, C. A.-F. (2004, 03). *In-vitro anti-inflammatory effect of Eucalyptus globulus and Thymus vulgaris: nitric oxide inhibition in J774A.1 murine macrophages.* Retrieved 01 22, 2015, from Pubmed: http://www.ncbi.nlm.nih.gov/pubmed/15005885

Wang GW1, Q. J. (2014, 03 14). *Inula sesquiterpenoids: structural diversity, cytotoxicity and anti-tumor activity.* Retrieved 01 23, 2015, from Pubmed: http://www.ncbi.nlm.nih.gov/pubmed/24387187

Worwood, V. A. (1993). *Aromantics.* Bantam Books.

Worwood, V. A. *The Fragrant Mind.* 1997: Bantam.

Yang H1, K. T. (2012, 09 22). *Analysis of the effects of essential oils on airborne bacteria in a customized bio-clean room.* Retrieved 01 21, 2015, from Pub med: http://www.ncbi.nlm.nih.gov/pubmed/22751732

Young, R. T. (2013). Cassia. In R. T. Young, *Essential Oil Safety for Health Professionals* (pp. (Kindle Locations 15332-15410). Guide for Health Care Professionals (Kindle Locations 17489-17528). Elsevier Health Sciences UK. Kindle Edition.

Young, T. a. (2013). Eucalyptus. In R. T. Young, *Essential Oil Safety for Health Professionals* (pp. (Kindle Locations 17489-17528).). Elsevier Health Sciences UK. Kindle Edition. .

Zhao CZ1, W. Y. (2008). *Effect of Spearmint oil on inflammation, oxidative alteration and Nrf2 expression in lung tissue of COPD rats.* Retrieved 01 15, 2015, from Pubmed: http://www.ncbi.nlm.nih.gov/pubmed/18705008

Zhou XM, Z. Y. (2012). *preventive-effects-of-citrus-reticulata-essential-oil-on-bleomycin-induced-pulmonary-fibrosis-in-rats-and-the-mechanism/*. Retrieved 01 15, 2015, from Journal of Chinese Integrative Medicine: http://aromaticscience.com/preventive-effects-of-citrus-reticulata-essential-oil-on-bleomycin-induced-pulmonary-fibrosis-in-rats-and-the-mechanism/

Disclaimer

by SEQ Legal

(1) Introduction

This disclaimer governs the use of this book. [By using this book, you accept this disclaimer in full. / We will ask you to agree to this disclaimer before you can access the book.]

(2) Credit

This disclaimer was created using an SEQ Legal template.

(3) No advice

The book contains information about aromatherapy and the use of essential oils. The information is not advice, and should not be treated as such.

[You must not rely on the information in the book as an alternative to qualified medical advice from a health professional. advice from an appropriately qualified professional. If you have any specific questions about any medical matter you should consult an appropriately qualified professional.]

[If you think you may be suffering from any medical condition you should seek immediate medical attention. You should never delay seeking medical advice, disregard medical advice, or discontinue medical treatment because of information in the book.]

(4) No representations or warranties

To the maximum extent permitted by applicable law and subject to section 6 below, we exclude all representations, warranties, undertakings and guarantees relating to the book.

Without prejudice to the generality of the foregoing paragraph, we do not represent, warrant, undertake or guarantee:

that the information in the book is correct, accurate, complete or non-misleading;

that the use of the guidance in the book will lead to any particular outcome or result; or

in particular, that by using the guidance in the book you will heal disease or work in any way as a cure for illness.

(5) Limitations and exclusions of liability

The limitations and exclusions of liability set out in this section and elsewhere in this disclaimer: are subject to section 6 below; and govern all liabilities arising under the disclaimer or in relation to the book, including liabilities arising in contract, in tort (including negligence) and for breach of statutory duty.

We will not be liable to you in respect of any losses arising out of any event or events beyond our reasonable control.

We will not be liable to you in respect of any business losses, including without limitation loss of or damage to profits, income, revenue, use, production, anticipated savings, business, contracts, commercial opportunities or goodwill.

We will not be liable to you in respect of any loss or corruption of any data, database or software.

We will not be liable to you in respect of any special, indirect or consequential loss or damage.

(6) Exceptions

Nothing in this disclaimer shall: limit or exclude our liability for death or personal injury resulting from negligence; limit or exclude our liability for fraud or fraudulent misrepresentation; limit any of our liabilities in any way that is not permitted under applicable law; or exclude any of our liabilities that may not be excluded under applicable law.

(7) Severability

If a section of this disclaimer is determined by any court or other competent authority to be unlawful and/or unenforceable, the other sections of this disclaimer continue in effect.

If any unlawful and/or unenforceable section would be lawful or enforceable if part of it were deleted, that part will be deemed to be deleted, and the rest of the section will continue in effect.

(8) Law and jurisdiction

This disclaimer will be governed by and construed in accordance with English law, and any disputes relating to this disclaimer will be subject to the exclusive jurisdiction of the courts of England and Wales.

(9) Our details

In this disclaimer, "we" means (and "us" and "our" refer to) *Build Your Own Reality* of SY8 1LQ.

9543579R00103

Printed in Great Britain
by Amazon.co.uk, Ltd.,
Marston Gate.